Sexual Beginnings

Sexual Beginnings

A Blueprint for Life

A Key to Harmonious Adult Relationships

Mary Vaughan Lindsey

iUniverse, Inc.
New York Lincoln Shanghai

Sexual Beginnings
A Blueprint for Life

Copyright © 2006 by Mary Vaughan Lindsey

iUniverse books may be ordered through booksellers or by contacting:

iUniverse
2021 Pine Lake Road, Suite 100
Lincoln, NE 68512
www.iuniverse.com
1-800-Authors (1-800-288-4677)

ISBN-13: 978-0-595-39337-4 (pbk)
ISBN-13: 978-0-595-83734-2 (ebk)
ISBN-10: 0-595-39337-3 (pbk)
ISBN-10: 0-595-83734-4 (ebk)

Printed in the United States of America

For All Those Who Have Loved Me

Acknowledgment

This book began in the mind and hearts of the author and Dr. Thomas Mazur who was then Director of Psychoendocrinology at Children's Hospital in Buffalo, New York. The impetus was our common desire to help parents nurture and educate their children to a higher level of psychological health. We had both found in our counseling practices so many families struggling to understand their children's sexuality. I was further encouraged in my endeavors by Dr. Thomas Frantz, then Acting Dean of the Graduate Department of Counseling Psychology at SUNYAB.

Several other editors such as Adele O'Connell, Pam Howell, Cathy Vaughan, Maureen Straight and Theresa Vaughan were all helpful in shaping my original manuscript into the finished product. Lee Vaughan proved to be proofreader *par excellence*.

Tom, Jim and Peggy Vaughan walked me through the necessary computer intricacies without, I might say, leaving a trace of skill. Tom helped me over the final hurdles from my first manuscript to its present form.

My two families—Vaughan and Lindsey—gave me love and encouragement in a thousand ways. I am very grateful.

And lastly, we all must give particular thanks to Gabrielle who at six months of age supervised our efforts, sitting gracefully like a little princess on the Grand Island office floor where we worked.

It is fair to say that this book could not have been birthed without the efforts of these labor coaches.

Table of Contents

List of Illustrations

Chapter 5

Chapter 6

Chapter 8

Chapter 9

Chapter 10

Chapter 11

Chapter 12

List of Tables

Section I

Male And Female, They Were Created

Chapter 1

The Relationship Connection

By degrees, however, my experience and personal reflection brought me…to the realization that the world would never be better and men (and women) happier until human beings learned to open their hearts, and put greater warmth and love into their relationships.

Ignace Lepp,[1]

My husband, Bob, finally succumbed to his four-year battle with cancer a year after our eldest son was married. In the following year, the newlyweds visited me often in an effort to assuage my loneliness. On one of their visits they announced the happy news of a coming baby. They were delighted and so was I. In my excitement I blurted out, "Oh, it will be a boy and he will be born on Bob's birthday." This was no premonition. I had no forethought of such an announcement—how could I know it was a boy and when he would be born? It was laughed off as a grandmotherly wish.

After they left, in spite of my elation at the good news, my heart was feeling great sadness that my husband would not share in watching his grandchildren grow. The due date for the baby came and went. The morning of my husband's birthday arrived. I awoke from a sound sleep at four am that morning, with the positive knowledge that my daughter-in-law was about to give birth. I prayed that all would be well with her and my son and the new little one.

At seven that evening my son was on the telephone to announce they were the proud parents of a baby boy! I asked, "What time did labor begin?" He replied, "About four o'clock this morning." A marvelous birthday gift for my husband! I realized then that Bob was sharing in my joy and that we were still connected—in a new and very special relationship—a relationship of the spirit.

Relationships are our connection to one another. In fact, all life is relational. Human beings are related to all other life from the genesis of the first cell. Trees and plants provide us with the air we breathe—our very lifeline. Animals and plants provide us with food, and from early civilization, shelter. The earth gives up its rich oil and minerals so we can survive. We look to past generations for ideas to build upon. Astronomers and astronauts search the skies to determine our future. All life is precious and interdependent.

A very beautiful description of our relationship to every living thing is given by Joyce Rupp, OSM. She calls it a melody of a cosmic dance.

> But the most astounding discovery that both awakened and affirmed my early childhood awareness is the fact that I am part of a vast and marvelous dance that goes on unceasingly at every moment in the most minute particles of the universe. Scientists tell us that these tiny parts of matter are always moving and intermingling with everything around them. I picture these invisible particles that compose every piece of existence as having little dancing feet. Something as sturdy as a boulder does its own boulder dance, but it also weaves in and out of the dance of the soil, the dance of the worm, the dance of the world. The stone, the soil, the worm, the wolf cannot be contained. They dance with everything else that is. What a marvel to

think that each cell of my body is part of an intricate interweaving of the dynamic life of creation![2]

In contrast to this deep interdependence with all the earth, people can be related incidentally or by choice—by circumstances such as work—through associations in neighborhoods and schools. We can be related more intimately through birth or through friendship.

Consider too, there is a relational order in our very being. First, we are related to God (or a Higher Power of your own belief) since God is the author of life. We are related in a very special manner to our parents, physically through the union of their ovum and sperm—and emotionally through their love for one another—the love that provides the required environment for healthy development. As our relationship to siblings and friends develop, we add another dimension to our being. We become a family. Becoming a family is the relationship that prepares us to establish a connection to our community, to our government and eventually to our world.

For each individual on this planet, relationships begin in the womb or even before that in the relationship of the parents. Who we are and how we relate to one another is a product of how we begin life. It is important whether we are welcomed or rejected, partially or otherwise. Maturity as an adult grows out of our early relationships. Whether for better or worse, the manner in which men and women relate to one another in any arrangements that brings forth a child influences our future—and so it continues—generation after generation.

Every relationship has a biological, psychological and spiritual component. We understand the origin of our biological and psychological beginnings, but what of the spirit? Science has been able to create a form of life, using the ova and sperm of an already living person. To actually create life—another human being—a unique individual—speaks of a creative love unequalled by human love. So we might say that life comes from Pure Love—a love that is beyond human capacity to duplicate but is reflected in our spirit.

It is my belief that each developing embryo in the womb as it grows remembers that Love on a primitive, non-verbal level. As the embryo grows and develops, is birthed and grows to maturity, is it that Pure Love that we restlessly seek in relationships. It is only when we return to that Love at the end of life that we attain full peace.

So to begin at the very beginning, we might say that life created by the union of man and woman contains a spiritual capacity to love emanating from the Pure Love it has already experienced. That capacity has to be respected and nurtured during life in the womb and after birth so that the knowledge of Pure Love is not lost.

As the Psalmist sings,

> You created every part of me: You put me together in my mother's womb,
> You saw my bones being formed, carefully put together in my mother's womb
> When I was growing there in secret
> You saw me before I was born (Psalm 139 (13-16)

We live in a violent, volatile world that has great need of improved relationships. The tragic loss of life on September 11, 2001 at the World Trade Center has extended our need to form relationships to a global level: relationships that involve fundamental differences of religion, cultural customs, personal preferences, dreams and goals. Our new world requires we become adept at reconciling these differences and forging peaceful relationships. As the author, James Carroll puts it: "relationship...is at the heart of human hope...community is the antidote to human woundedness."[3]

How wounded is our society? We will consider in the next chapter how relationships have become broken.

Chapter 1—Endnotes

1 Lepp, Ignace, *The Psychology of Loving*, Helicon, Baltimore, 1963

2 Rupp, Joyce, OSM, *The Dance of Life*, St. Anthony Messenger, May 2002, p 36

3 Carroll, James, *Constantine's Sword*, Paulist Press, New York, NY, 2001

Chapter 2

Society Today

The primary law which operates in all human societies
and governs their culture in any location or
environment is the past and present method
of regulating the relations between the sexes.

John Unwin,[1]

In our present volatile world, nations are seeking ways to avoid nuclear war, to prevent genocide and provide for the hungry, ill and homeless of the world. Can we be successful at the global level if we fail to establish harmonious relationships at the individual level? To help our children learn to be peaceful, we need to provide them with a peaceful environment in which to grow.

Common sense tell us each generation influences the next generation and as Dr. Unwin concludes, peaceful relations between the sexes are primary to providing the next generation with a less hostile world.

Present statistics tell us very clearly we have not reached the establishment of peaceful relationships on the individual level:

* ❖ 51% of marriages end in divorce, the highest rate among industrial nations

* ❖ Domestic violence in the state of Florida alone resulted in 321 homicides in one year[2]

* ❖ More than 25,000 Americans are murdered each year, making homicide the 10th leading cause of death according to the 1993 APA report

* ❖ In a survey of 8000 men and 8000 women made by the National Institute of Justice, the Institute estimates that approximately 1.5 million American women and more than 800,000 men are raped or assaulted by an intimate partner annually[3]

* ❖ Teenagers are 21/2 times more likely to be victims of violent crimes. Interpersonal violence occurs most frequently among peers at school, family members or people of the same social circles

* ❖ One out of 4 girls and one out of 19 boys will be abused before they reach the age of eighteen

* ❖ 8 and 10-year olds are committing adult crimes—children perform rape and murder before their adult years

* ❖ Newborns are being killed by their young parents[4]

Dean Ornish, in his latest book entitled *Love and Survival, the Scientific Basis for the Healing Power of Intimacy*, pinpoints that the real epidemic in our culture is an emotional and spiritual disease of the heart caused by a profound sense of loneliness and isolation. Is this further evidence that we have lost the skill to form harmonious relationships?

The capacity for nurturing one another grows best in the fertile soil of mature, loving parents. Too often we assume maturity is a matter of age—legally a person is considered an adult at age twenty-one. Actually, few of us attain maturity. It is a slow journey from conception on through life, governed and enhanced by genes, hormones and environment—especially the family environment. The ideal environment of two loving parents cannot be replaced in the development of infants. Each step of development from conception to adulthood is a natural maturation process which we need to respect, a process which must be allowed to develop at its own pace with supportive love.

Science is teaching us daily in many new ways that a mature identity as a male or female begins in the womb and there is a natural progression from embryo to adulthood. This knowledge should lead us to cooperate with nature rather than frustrate it; to facilitate the natural stages of growth rather than ignore them.

We know a great deal about child development but frequently parents unknowingly frustrate this natural development from their own lack of awareness. Awareness of a body of knowledge permeates a culture very slowly as people have to be persuaded in order to change and old beliefs die hard. Very often it is economic pressure that dictates a parent's response to their children. Busy, harried parents have little time or energy for nurturing. We all need cultural support—both in our own development toward maturity in relationships of all kinds and in guiding our children.

Whatever the reason for the break-up of relationships, family violence and/or national loneliness and isolation, all parents should be aware of the following:

❖ We do know with certainty that the earliest critical period in our natural development is from conception to three.

❖ The greatest period of our physical growth and brain development is from conception to three.

❖ Our sense of the world begins in the period of conception to three.

❖ Our sense of gender identity and self-worth begins in the period of conception to age three approximately, depending on the child and the parents.

What greater knowledge do we need to convince us as a society to provide cultural assurance that parents and children are together in a health-giving environment during these early years? It is not only the job of parents. It is for all of us to provide such a vital living space. Other nations are providing for such togetherness—why can't we?

Unfortunately, we will attempt to *fix* the *problem* after the fact with programs on how to *develop* intimacy. Granted we need present help for those of us who are striving for a balanced relationship. However, we need to prevent the condition of isolation and the inability to effect an intimate relationship from beginning in the first place.

To understand more clearly how our culture needs to change, the following pages will trace the journey from conception to three years, relating such a journey to adult sexual identity and maturity;—the importance of early childhood events in forming a basis for harmonious relations between the sexes;—how early prevention can lessen crime, violence and suicide in our nation.

The statistics we quoted at the beginning of the chapter merely outline the perimeter of the difficulty we have with harmonious relationships. They only convey limited information. Let's consider the actual words of one of these numbers—an individual mother—a single parent.

Chapter 2—Endnotes

1   John Unwin, *Sex and Culture*, Oxford U Press, London, England, 1934

2   AP News Report, *Sun Herald*, Orlando, FL 3/14, 1998

3   AP News report, *Daily Gazette* 7/14/2000

4   Lloyd J. Thomas, PHD, Psychologist, *Daily Gazette*, 4/12/02

Chapter 3

Parents As Environment

The high calling of parenthood must be more adequately
recognized, respected and honored by our Society.
Therein lies the future of our Nation

National Council of Juvenile and Family Court Judges[1]

Sexuality is not a separate compartment of human life,
it is a radiance pervading every human relationship,
but assuming a particular intensity at certain points

Alan Watts, *Nature, Man and Woman*[2]

In his work *The Youngest Parents*, Robert Coles relates how a 15-year old girl with a one-year old daughter tells of her experience:

> I think I let myself get pregnant—that's what I now have discovered. I could have prevented it from happening, but I had nothing else to look forward to doing, and so this baby of mine was my one and only hope. The trouble is, if you're not becoming anyone yourself, then you're not going to be much of a mother—mean, you'll rise and fall with every little good or bad moment, because there's no life you have, other than waiting on the baby and that's not good for either of you![3]

What insight for a fifteen-year-old teenager! How can we teach our children to have such wisdom before the need for teenage choices that chart their course for the rest of their lives? A counselor, who guided me on many personal decisions, once told me that we can't put an old head on young shoulders. I hear the wisdom of that saying. On the other hand, what tools are we giving our youngsters so that they can be "becoming anyone" and are able to form the next generation?

I believe the fifteen-year old used the term "becoming anyone yourself" as her way of expressing a need for a self-identity. Self-identity is an often-used term but what do we mean by it?

Such a question has haunted me for a very long time. How do you answer it? One day my then college-age daughter, returning home from classes, entered the kitchen and without any preliminary words, asked me, "If someone asked you who you were, what would you answer?" Knowing she was not just asking for my name and address, I thought for a few moments before answering. "I am a child of God, a wife and a mother, and a person of integrity." "Bingo," she said. "Isn't it wonderful to know who you are, I wish I did!"

What led me to say those particular words? Obviously, they expressed a series of priorities in my life that were indelibly imprinted or I could not have come up with them in a few moments. In fact, I surprised myself.

What those categories seemed to express was my spirituality, my life's commitment and my self-worth. It was my "being anyone." For me these values begin with new life as early as in the womb and build throughout one's life. How important, then, that parents have their own sense of identity and are able to guide their children to maturity—so they, in turn, make good choices.

But parents cannot do it alone! Our culture needs an overhaul.

Parents are not able to spend sufficient time with their children in order to allow both to mature. The personal growth of the above-quoted young woman is evident in the mere one year she has spent with her baby.

Now that she has experienced intimacy in the form of mother love, I wonder what her criteria would be for entering into a second sexual relationship? How stable has her own sexual identity as a woman "becoming anyone" progressed? Does she value herself so that someone else sees her value? Probably not at present—but in her favor is her gift of self-reflection. Will she be able to get the right kind of societal support?

How do we encourage the development of masculine and feminine identity—the sense of "becoming anyone"? In the words of the former First Lady Hillary Clinton it does take a village because society must support the principles that lead each individual to a mature sense of self as a man or a woman. However, each child develops in a unique parental environment—which for better or worse helps to shape the identity of the adult person. Marital discord and rejection of pregnancy provide an environment that, like genes and chromosomes, can influence negatively the sexual identity of the child. Such influence, the same as genes and chromosomes, begins in the womb.

Babies establish, positively or otherwise, an intimate womb relationship with their mothers that needs to be continued until the child achieves a degree of individuation and a sense of gender, a sense of separateness from the parent, and a sense of being a boy or a girl. This relationship of mother-child, together with a bonding of mother-father-child, becomes the forerunner and foundation for all the child's future intimate relationships. A warm, loving environment in the womb and after birth fosters a capacity for the development of a level of trust, a degree of autonomy, and self-identity for the infant. These three elements are vital to the development of the child. It is also vital that they first be developed in the period that spans from conception to approximately three years of age—the first of several *critical periods* for the formation of sexual identity.

More than one-half our children are being parented by single women. What does that say for our future? This is not a criticism of single parents—many of them do a superb job—but nature intended parenting to be a two-parent labor of love.

A recent Australian study involving 10,641 people contradicts the notion that marriage emotionally oppresses women—an idea put forth by feminist scholar, Jessie Bernard about thirty years ago. The study found mental illness to be equal (16%) in both men and women. Divorced people fared the worst with 25% of both sexes suffering emotional problems. Single persons fared slightly better at 22% of women and 26% of men afflicted with mental disorders. Married people were best off with only 13% of both sexes suffering from emotional disorders.[4]

Most of us enter marriage unprepared. We might think we are prepared, especially intellectually, but it is only in the living of a marriage that we can know of its joys and pitfalls. 51% of marriages fail! Can we as a nation accept this failure? And what would correcting it demand of us?

The meeting of men and women on an equal basis—so necessary in the process of finding our identity and allowing others to have theirs—is placed in difficulty if we place our primary value on the physical (erotic) aspect of sexuality. Relationships are frequently built on sexual interaction, with both parties wishing for more than the physical expression of their love. It is very difficult to sustain any relationship, sexual or otherwise, and recognize each partner's equality. The Joyces tersely phrase the difficulty: "The idea of fundamental differences within the idea of fundamental equality."[5] Intimacy grows as we manage to incorporate this basic profound idea into our relationships.

Though men and women are equal, they are different in the very depth of their existence. To be real about this truth is what makes marriage so difficult. We enter marriage expecting complete understanding and companionship as a matter of course, rather than a life-long quest to be sought after. Part of the accent on sexual prowess and the thrust of women's lib to enter into heretofore male realms may be due to the fact that society does not value the quiet simplicity of nurturing love in either men or women. So women strive for recognition in masculine ways in an effort to establish their own identity, failing to realize the worth of their own life-giving qualities and their intuitive method of thinking.

Marriages might last longer and the divorce rate be reduced if men and women respected the mystery of their singular identities and enjoyed and encouraged the differences.

Marriage is the graduate school training for mature adulthood. Through a loving union and the birth of a child we gradually come to the concept of unconditional love. When two people commit themselves to marriage and experience true love, there is a real desire to share the beauty of that love. Mutual admiration is not enough. Three at least are needed before love can be perfected. Love needs to be shared. In that sense, a child perfects the love of parents. The love that joins any two equal individuals is in itself something so good, so precious that it must be shared with another. Love multiples while it unifies. This is the environment in which a child should ideally be conceived and birthed. The love that flows from one to another in this threesome will influence the growth of identity of each of them.

Individualism has become of the mantra of Americans and has influenced our views on marriage. We no longer consider marriage a necessity for parenthood or relationships. Gradually though, there seems to be an awakening to the possibility that committed marriage could help to develop our children into healthy adults. In addition, the importance to our nation of the idea of commitment on the part of the community is slowly being recognized. Marriage is the first community and it is important that each member be nurtured in love so that the process of communal relationships is begun first with sharing with each other and their child, then gradually reaching out further to the broader community.

It is a present-day axiom that in order to give love, one has to first love oneself. However, a sense of self-worth is not acquired externally. It is seeded at the very beginning of life in the womb when a nurturing environment encourages growth. It is an innate sense developed from the loving welcome from mature parents who are committed to the task.

As Thomas Moore describes it: "This self is not something to be fabricated by achievement, cleverness, training, or learning. It is not the product of self-analysis or understanding. It is a gift, waiting to be accepted and nurtured in its unfolding."[6]

Chapter 3—Endnotes

[1] National Council of Juvenile and Family Court Judges,1989, Report of the CaliforniaTask Force on Self-esteem, 1990, published by the Chamber of Commerce of California.

[2] Watts, Alan, *Nature, Man and Woman*, Pantheon Press, New York, New York, 1958

[3] Coles, Robert, *The Youngest Parents: Teenage Pregnancy As It Shapes Lives*, Center for Documentary Studies in association with WW Norton & Company, NY & London, 1997

[4] DeVaus, David, LaTrobe University in Melbourne, Australia, reported by AP in *The Daily Gazette*, 10/5/02

[5] Joyce, Robert and Mary, *New Dimensions in Sexual Love*. St. John's University Press. Collegeville, MN. 1970

[6] Moore, Thomas, *Original Self*, Harper-Collins, New York, NY 2000

Chapter 4

Society As Environment

Each society evolves a particular view about the genesis of life and death that harmonizes with its total philosophy and organization, which then determines cultural attitudes and myths and behavior in relation to childbearing. The philosophy and the behavioral patterns become woven together, creating a society which then influences the next generation. Each society thus has characteristic effects on the environment of the womb from the earliest moments of development

Leni Schwartz, *The World of the Unborn*[1]

A true story about Patty and Ed illustrates one of our society's "characteristic effects" on the "environment of the womb" as described in the foregoing quote by Leni Schwartz.

Patty and Ed, two college seniors from a midwestern city, came to the Mental Health Center for advice. Both had been brought up in traditionally religious, middle-class families. However, their sex life was separate and apart from their beliefs. It was based on the needs of both. For Ed, their relationship was a way to have regular and easily available sex. For Patty, it was a means of getting the love and approval that she so desperately sought. In counseling sessions with Patty alone, we found that such affirmation and approval had been denied her by her mother who constantly found fault with her and who had taught her the concept of a punishing God. When Patty became pregnant, she and Ed viewed the situation very differently. Initially, Patty accepted her pregnancy even though it interfered with her plans to graduate that year. It was kind of exciting to have a baby—someone to love—and to love her. Besides, she really believed Ed would feel the same.

Ed, however, viewed the pregnancy as a surefire way of being "trapped poor." He was in no financial state to care for a family. He wanted a chance to form a career. He offered to pay for an abortion and even expressed a willingness to marry Patty, but adamantly refused to provide for the child if Patty carried it to full term. Patty was three months into her pregnancy. In her mind, she was being asked to choose between losing her child or losing her boyfriend—between a "love" she felt she knew and one she could only hope for. And then—there were these nagging thoughts…was it right to get an abortion…wasn't that taking a life? Well…she would put these thoughts aside for now. Ed was important to her…besides, he was right…they didn't have any money.…

It is obvious Patty and Ed's relationship based on their needs had met an impasse.

Whose needs will prevail? Would they ever be able to develop a truly loving relationship? Each couple has to find their own solution. It is a common situation found over and over again in all our cities everyday. According to the incoming president of American College of Obstetricians,[2] half of all US pregnancies or about three million yearly are unintended and more than a million of them end in abortion.

It brings to mind Mari Evans' poem:

> If there be sorrow
> let it be for things undone
> undreamed
> unrealized

unattained,
to these add one:
love withheld
restrained.[3]

However, in this book we cannot solve Patty and Ed's dilemma. This book is about what is taking place with Patty and Ed's baby. Society has a wealth of information to help Patty with her pregnancy but much of it is ignored and some of it never reaches the women who are pregnant. What chance does this child have for a warm welcome if they decide to keep the baby?

In the past decade it is true that more help is being given to unwed mothers and there are more parenting classes for two-parent families. However, the culture to which we bring newborns is anti-children.

As Americans we are proud of our freedoms—freedom of religion—freedom of speech—freedom to choose many of the necessities of life such as education, type of employment—how we spend our leisure. However, there is always the other side of the coin. With freedom comes the responsibility to preserve it and that includes preserving the freedom of the other person.

Presently, according to statistics earlier quoted, our society is tending toward violence and a disregard for the rights of others. How can we stop that trend and inject the next generation with a nonviolent sense of themselves and a regard for others?

We have to start at the beginning—with the care and nurture of our children. Our laws must reflect that care and the whole nation has to be involved. Suggestions for how we might accomplish such a change will be dealt with in a later chapter. For now, let us consider the basic need brought about by the very skill and ingenuity for which Americans are noted. As I see it, technology and the profit motive have taken precedence over our sense of responsibility for the common good. Our laws are beginning to foreshadow big brother in an effort to protect our individual desires. Reproductive technology has grown to a skill level beyond our consideration of the ethics involved. Careers have supplanted time for family togetherness and growth.

We allow television and the internet to teach values to our children as we deny them our presence and intimate guidance in a world of growing complexity. We are telling our children that the parent-child relationship is based on how much material satisfaction we can provide. Implicitly we teach them that our family bond—mother-father-child—is unimportant.

If our society were truly interested in caring for the young, we would provide:

❖ Paid family leave
❖ Mandated parent education

❖ Improved, affordable health care

❖ School health clinics, well-staffed and connected with a health-based institution

❖ Improving community awareness that marriage has been found to be the key social institution for bringing up healthy, happy, competent children

To educate the community, more debates about family issues should take place on a national level. A use of television with the same amount of hype that we give to war news and reports of violence would be effective. Sylvia Ann Hewlitt poses an excellent question for debate: "The differential sacrifices women make in comparison to men, the need to think about those sacrifices and to plan around them, even the need to think about the whole issue of blending family and career life."[4]

We also need to research why reported violence among intimates[5] is so widespread even though at least one-quarter of the physical attacks are not reported. The joint survey of the Justice Department and Centers for Disease Control revealed 1.5 percent of women and 0.9 percent of men said they were raped or physically assaulted by their partner in the last twelve months.

A report by *Child Trends* revealed, based on a survey of 8000 young people ages 12 to 16, that teens surveyed in 2000 said they first had sex at their family's home. The report also cited that by the time students are in the ninth grade, 34 percent have had sexual intercourse. That rises to 60 percent by 12th grade. On the other hand researchers also reported that teen girls who are close to their moms are more likely to stay virgins.[6]

Early sexual interaction not only gives rise to an increase in unwed mothers giving birth. It misuses the precious time of adolescence—substituting early gratification for mature growth.

Research is now showing that couples who don't live together before marriage, have a better shot at staying together as do those whose parents stay married. Present television programs would be helpful to make this finding known to the general public. Just spot announcements by the studio would help to get the news out.

Medco Health Solutions, a NJ-based pharmacy benefits manager, reports a 28 percent rate of growth for prescription drugs for those youths under 19 years of age.[7] To further emphasize the need for improved health care, the *New England Journal of Medicine* issued a report that while genes play a part in the risk of cancer, (about 30 percent on average), the rest of the cancer risk was influenced by environmental factors such as experiences in the womb, one's upbringing and smoking and drinking habits.[8]

And who will care for the orphans created by the AIDS crisis? At the recent International Aids Conference (Barcelona Spain—7/11/02) attendees were told that by 2001, 13.4 million children had lost one or both parents to AIDS. It was estimated that by 2010 the toll will pass 25 million.

I believe that parents have a tremendous influence on our cultural values. They have the power to determine the survival of the human race. Failure to recognize and use that power demeans our society. It is not enough to birth children—we must be culturally responsible for them. As Erikson reminds us, all leaders of society begin as children.[9]

How we nurture our children will determine both our future and theirs in this violent world.

Chapter 4—Endnotes

1   Schwartz, Leni, *The World of the Unborn* Richard Publishers, New York, NY, 1980

2   American College of Obstetricians, Annual Meeting *Daily Gazette* 5/1/01

3   Evans, Mari, *Maryknoll*, July 1981—p.33

4   Quote from Commencement address by Wm. Raspberry at UNC at Chapel Hill, NC—reported in D*aily Gazette* 6/17/02

5   Julie Samuels, National Institute of Justice Survey with Center for Disease Control, *AP report* 7/14/02

6   Brown, Sarah, Director National Campaign to Prevent Teen Pregnancy, AP News Report, *Daily Gazette* 9/26/02

7   Medco Health, AP report, *Daily Gazette*, 9/19/02

8   Dr. Robert N. Hoover, Director of Epidemiology and Biostatistics program at National Cancer Institute in Bethesda, Md., *Los Angeles Times*, 7/13/00

9   Erikson, Erik H., *Identity and the Life Cycle*, W.W. Norton & Co., New York, N.Y., 1959, 1980, 1994

Masculine And Feminine Identity Years 0-3

Chapter 5

The Infant's First World

A proper understanding of the origins of human nature and human diversity, then, rests on an understanding of these two fundamental features of organisms: (1) each organism is the subject of continuous development throughout its life; (2) the developing organism is at all times under the influence of mutually interacting genes and environment.

Richard Lewontin[1]

Biology experts tells us we never cease to develop and change throughout our lifetime. What form that development takes is a result of the interaction of genes and environment. Our environment would include the immediate environment—our parents, their health and relationship; cultural trends of the generation of which we are a part; and laws, customs and traditions of the country of which we are citizens.

In the infant's first world, the immediate environment is the mother's womb. As all pregnant women do, Patty, the college student referred to in the preceding chapter, brings to that beginning of life three essential aspects of nourishment. Her body feeds the body of the infant, while creating an emotional climate in which the spirit of the child can develop. The environment of the womb, science had made clear to us, is defined and controlled by the physical health and behavioral habits of the mother-to-be.

What is less studied by many scientists and less popularly known is that the environment of the womb is affected by the emotional well-being of the mother and the adult psychological health and knowledge of both father and mother. In other words, the relationship between parents and child does not begin at birth, but is established while the child is developing in the womb. Further, the preceding and ongoing marital relationship of the parents has an effect on the environment of the womb. Patty and Ed have not been able to commit themselves to a love deep enough to encompass the little one they have created. They have not evolved from self-love sufficiently to allow them to form a strong union that could reach out to another.

Can the fetus experience their lack of welcome—the mother's anxiety—the father's rejection? We can't know for certain. What is certain is that before a newborn infant has a sense of self, s/he must interact with his/her environment. His/her environment is the physical condition of the womb, which in turn is affected by the mother's environment. Acceptance of the condition of pregnancy and a healthy womb promote the development of the fetus. That is nature's plan. Such interaction begins in the womb between mother and fetus and continues until birth and beyond.

From such interaction the infant incorporates within its developing self, on a primitive level, a sense of gender. Genes alone do not convey gender. Developing a sense of being masculine or feminine is a complex process that evolves with the infant's biological/neurological beginnings, plus a psychological component from his/her relationship with parents, and the freedom of his/her spiritual uniqueness. Before an infant can learn to express any response verbally, s/he understands a great deal from primitive non-verbal impressions of what kind of world this is and who his/her parents are—if they are loving and if s/he is lovable. Parents are often unaware of their child's sensitive recording of such impressions. These impressions form the basis of advice to parents to speak to the beginning life in the womb—to use massage to let the infant know of their love. Babies can benefit from stimulation as early as the third month of pregnancy, at which point they primitively perceive spatial orientation and tactile stimuli.

This critical time in the womb is the beginning of a sense of self. Without nurturing interaction, both physically and psychologically, an opportunity is lost to establish a firm foundation for his/her inner sense of masculinity and femininity and a sense of self-worth.

Elizabeth Noble, author of Primal Connections, reminds us:

> Unconditional love is a difficult ideal. It is hard for people to give what they didn't get and when the unconditional love and nurturing of uterine environment is lacking, it is difficult for the offspring to provide it for the next generation.[2]

The three factors that are most critical to a psychologically and physically healthy pregnancy are:

1) a desire for the child

2) the quality of the relationship between the parents and,

3) the physical and psychological health of the parents

These three factors do not act independently of one another but are intertwined in a complex fashion to form the environment of the womb. If one of these factors is awry, the spirit of the developing infant can be wounded before birth by a sense of rejection even though apparently physically healthy.

Lewonton, the popular geneticist maintains: "History begins with the moment of conception."[3] I would like the reader to consider that at conception, life (the history of the individual) begins as a three segment developmental process—physical, psychological and spiritual.

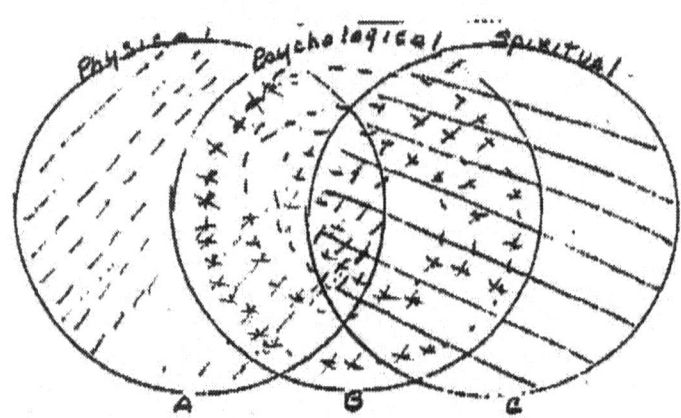

Figure 5-1 Physical, Psychological and Spiritual Beginnings of Life—Straight.

When the chromosomes of the sperm and the egg meet (sperm from the male and the egg from the female) they form one cell—a new individual. In the nucleus of that cell is contained all the instructions needed to build an organism as complex as a human being. For this one cell to develop into a baby, three areas influence its growth. The ideal womb environment requires:

A) physical wellness—appropriate hygiene, diet, exercise, rest, recreation for both parents but especially the mother

B) healthy mental and emotional climate—ideally created by two receptive, knowledgeable and willing parents

C) spiritual maturity—unconditional love

Each process is inextricably linked to the other two, and although discrete statements can validly be made about each facet of development, they cannot be considered as entirely separate. We are holistic beings who can be studied in small segments but researchers[4] recognize that any one segment is part of the whole, the components of which cannot be fully understood in isolation. It follows then that all three components are a part of and important to the formation of our individual identity as male or female. This complex, intertwined interaction continues throughout life. Serious neglect of one of these facets of development at any point in time impairs all three.

Keith Moore in his book *The Developing Human*, offers the following definition:

Development is a continuous process that begins when an ovum is fertilized by the sperm and ends in death. It is a process of growth and differentiation which transforms a single cell into a multicellular adult human being. Most developmental changes occur during the embryonic and fetal period, but important changes also occur during infancy, childhood, adolescence and adulthood.[5]

The emphasis here, as you can see, is on development in the womb. The study of the embryonic and fetal period has progressed rapidly in recent years as our technology has allowed us to examine what is actually going on in a woman's womb. However, as in all new developments in science, there is disagreement as to the significance of the findings. For instance, controversy persists regarding the so-called causes of gender identity or sex differences. Is the primary determinant genes, hormones, or the social environment? The possibility seems very real that it is all three, with each component assuming a varying level of importance at various *critical* times of development.

At the risk of oversimplification, we will take a look at all three.

For a graphic illustration of the beginning of our unique sexuality, we can turn to Linnert Nilsson's beautiful photographs of the beginning of life that were published in *Life Magazine* (August 1990). Here we can actually see the unfertilized egg *communicating* with the sperm, selecting and encouraging the fittest.

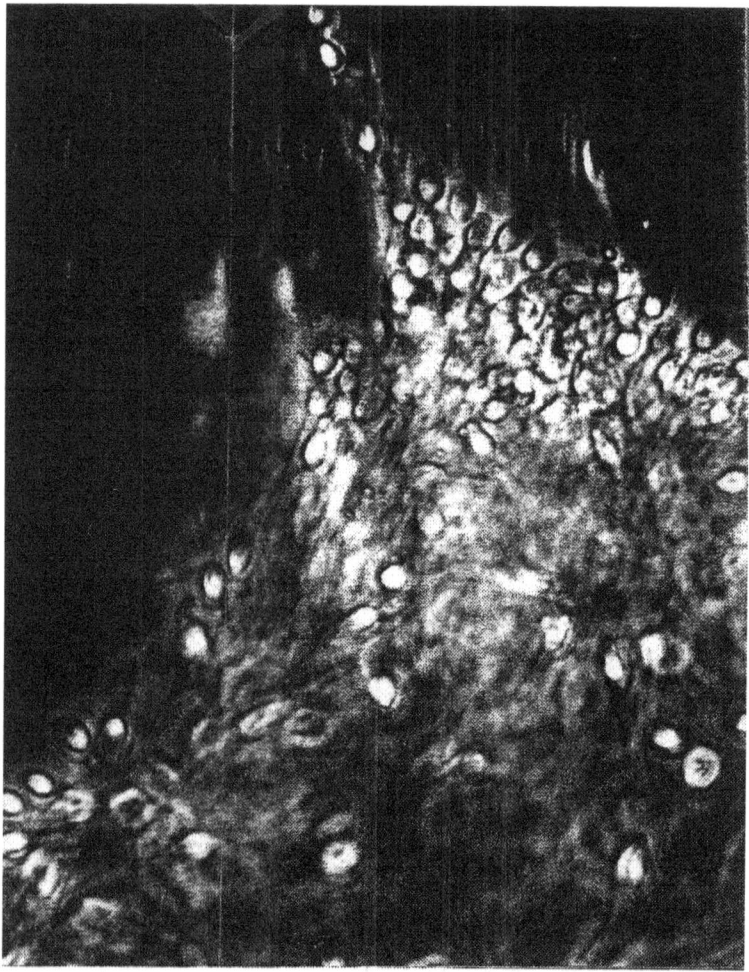

Figure 5-2 Although few will finish, about 250 million sperm start the five-to-seven-inch journey from the vagina to the uterus and then on to the fallopian tube, where once a month an egg may be waiting. In this photo, sperm attempt to penetrate the mucous plug at the cervix, the constricted opening to the uterus; only a fraction of the sperm may make it through a few channels no wider than a hair. Linnert Nilsson, The Worlds Within Our Bodies, *Life Magazine*, January 1970.

The sperm from the male and the ovum (egg) from the female unite and complete each other in one cell that has direction and movement and is capable of reproduction. A fertilized human egg has the capacity not only to develop into a baby, but to develop into an individual with brown eyes like his father or a chin like his grandmother. How is this fantastic progression accomplished?

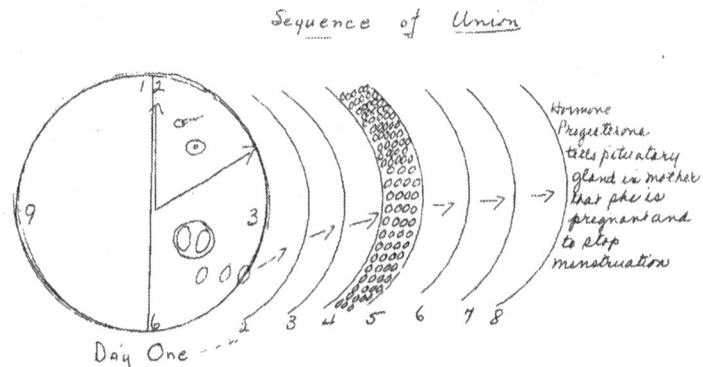

Figure 5-3 Sequence of Union—Straight

In 6 hours:	One sperm enters one ovum in the Fallopian tube; The ovum closes—sperm loses its tail Chromosomes draw irresistibly into a single nucleus that contains the blueprint for the individual.
In 12 hours	Cell splits into two and begins journey to womb; It multiplies into 100 cells before entering uterus
Within 4 days:	Cells settle into lining of the uterus
Within 8 days:	The hormone progesterone tells the pituitary gland in the mother that she is pregnant and to stop menstruation. The journey has begun!

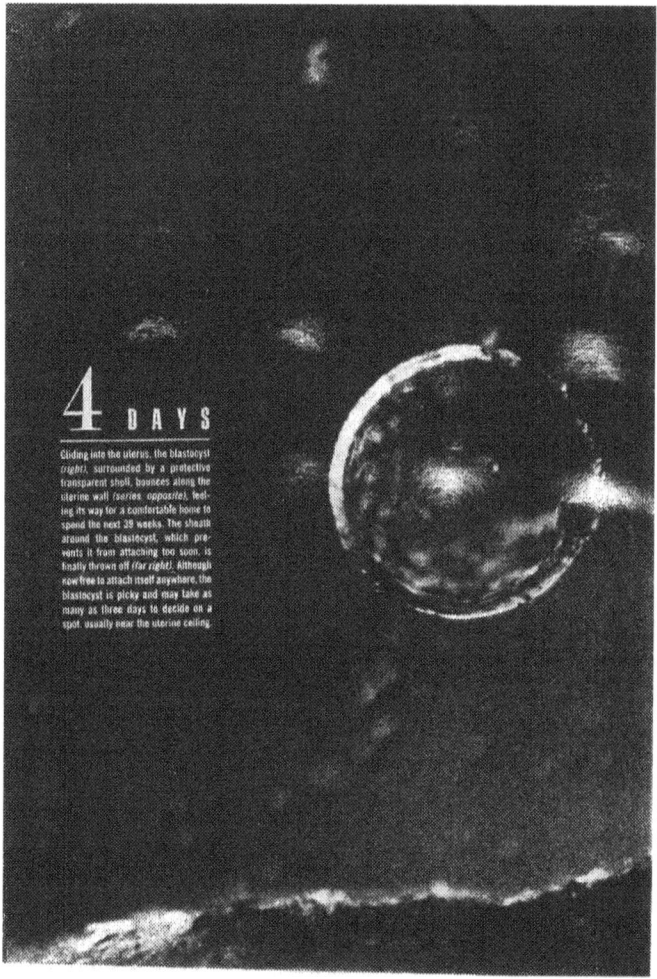

Figure 5-4 4 Days—Attachment to the Uterus Wall (Nilsson)

Chromosomes

Our bodies are composed of millions of cells, but we all begin our existence with the one cell to which both parents contribute as previously mentioned. Both of our parents had twenty-three pairs of chromosomes consisting of two members, one each received from the egg and the sperm of their parents. (A chromosome is a rodlike structure that carries the genes containing the code for our individual uniqueness.) What happens at conception is a miraculous transfer of

traits from both parents to a new life in a combination that can never be duplicated. Each new life is unique. What happens to this uniqueness (via genes and
chromosomes) during development in the womb helps to determine the identity
of the individual—not simply whether the infant is a boy or a girl, but different
degrees of sexual differentiation that may be at variance with our stereotypes of a
boy or a girl, but which, nevertheless contribute to that individual's uniqueness.

In both parents, the two members of each of twenty-two pairs of chromosomes are identical to each other. In women, the twenty-third pair (the sex chromosome) is made up of two identical members designated XX. In men, the
twenty-third chromosome (also the sex chromosome) has two different members,
one identical with that of the female X and one (a smaller one) called the Y chromosome (Figure 5-5).

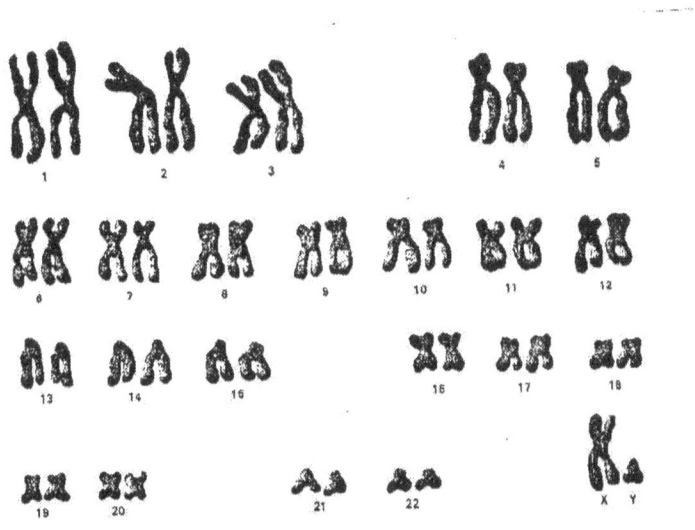

Figure 5-5 The 23 sets of chromosomes in a typical human cell. Note the similarity
between matched pairs. Note also the distinctive appearance of the X and Y chromosomes that determine sex. (from Krieger, The Human Reproductive System, Basic
Biology in Color Series, Vol. 4)

The one cell contributed to our beginning by our parents receives one member of each chromosome pair. Because the female chromosome has two X members, each new egg will contain an X chromosome. Half of the sperm cells will

contain an X member and half will contain the Y member. Therefore, as one would expect, an XX union of the egg and sperm will create a female and an XY union will create a male. However, it is not that simple. Logically, you would assume that the Y chromosome would be the male influence. What we find, however, is something very interesting.

Only the tiniest part of the Y chromosome is responsible for producing a boy instead of a girl, less than 0.1 percent, a single gene. Our latest finding is that this gene has instructions for making a molecule that acts as a switch to open for reading a series of other genes in the chromosome. The chemicals, for which those genes provide patterns, do all the rest of the work. Both sexes have all these other genes in the chromosome. The switch is all that is necessary to make a boy.

Yet, the Y chromosome has a definite effect because its absence creates abnormalities. XO people (those without Y chromosomes) are females who are infertile and have undeveloped ovaries. So it can be said that the Y chromosome pushes the fetus toward male development. Both sexes have X chromosomes, so there are no genes carried for *females only*. Males who have XX chromosomes are sterile. The X chromosome can be inherited from either the male or female parent. (Nature, as you might say, is showing equality of the sexes at the very beginning!) In the early development of the female, one of the X chromosomes becomes inactive. Sometimes the maternal inherited one is deactivated. Sometimes the paternal X chromosome becomes inactive.

Nature seems to be sending mixed messages. The mystery becomes a little clearer when you consider the presence of two X chromosomes' importance for girls even though one becomes deactivated as XO girls have imperfectly formed ovaries. XXY males are sterile. It is a very complex process that merits further study. With all the gene studies presently ongoing, an early resolution seems possible.

Genes

At this point you may ask: "Why all this fuss about which chromosome we inherit from which parent?" Remember that chromosomes carry genes. It is estimated that each cell contains approximately 30,000 genes. Genes are present on the initial chromosomes from the mother and father which make up the beginning cell of the individual and are duplicated in each cell as the cell divides and reproduces. Genes contain a set of chemical instruction for the embryo's development. Each gene sets out a program for the production of a single polypeptide (a protein compound); untold thousands of proteins give the human body its form and function.

Recent studies have identified the genes that act on the early embryo to lend it shape and pattern, transforming a nondescript comma of tissue into a human with limbs, fingers, brain, spinal cord and body shape.

Scientists at the present time are deeply involved in the study of genes. More information is beginning to be available as to how specific genes direct specific body development. However, myths about the influence of genes have already begun to be accepted. For instance, remarks such as, "Herbert is obese, but he can't help it—it's in his genes. He'll always be fat." Such a fatalistic view of the influence of genes is not valid. There can be extreme variability about how a gene is expressed, even within a family with the same genes. Environment also plays a role in this instance—nutrition, the type of work Herbert does, his work environment, the climate he lives in, his social experience and other factors may all contribute to Herbert's obesity. Just how some of these environmental factors influence an individual's development, will be dealt with in later chapters.

Presently, the general consensus among endocrinologists, biologists and researchers in various fields relating to fetal sexual development confirms the close interaction of genes, hormones and tissue environment at critical periods. Lewontin, quoted earlier, believes not only that organisms react variously to a particular stage in a particular environment, but that the effect of genes and environment cannot be separated. Genes and chromosomes may be said to respond to the environment provided for them in the womb, and this response in part determines the uniqueness of that individual.[6]

Hormones

Equal participants with genes and chromosomes in the development of an individual—especially in terms of sexual development—are the secretion of hormones. Hormones are chemicals, carried in the blood, which are produced by the ductless glands, principal among which is the pituitary gland. Hormones can have a great influence on the sex of the embryo during the early stages of development, sometimes modifying the sex already genetically determined.

Both male and female hormones, released by the ovaries or testes, have a general stimulating effect, causing increased cell division and growth. Very simply put, the sex hormones have two principal effects:

❖ to make the sexual organs (gonads) grow, and

❖ to stimulate the sexual organs so that they themselves secrete secondary sex hormones.

What we often don't realize is that the only difference between the hormones found in males and those found in females is one of proportion. The sex cells (gonads) in both males and females secrete the so-called female hormone estrogen. But females secrete more estrogen than do males. Hormones are not direct products of genes, but are synthesized by enzymes that are coded for by genes. Both sexes have active genes that code for these enzymes, but the mere presence of these enzymes will not cause sexual differentiation. Likewise, the mere presence of the hormone, no matter what its concentration, is not sufficient to cause sexual differentiation. Rather, the tissues involved must be receptive to the hormone. Again, this underscores the importance of the environment of the womb.

Testosterone, known as the male hormone (although it is also present in a lesser amount in the female) generally allows the male fetus to develop male genitalia and male internal reproductive organs. If testosterone is not available at the critical time, the fetus develops into a female. There are possible variations in this process, however, and sometimes nature fails and the developing infant's outward genitalia do not correspond with its internal reproductive organs It is easier to accept the great variations possible in individual sexuality when we understand the variation in mother's and infant's hormone levels and the unique environment of each womb.

In normal development, during the first quarter of fetal development, male and female look very much alike. The same sex gland and genital primordia are formed in both sexes. From then on, in normal development, sex chromosomal, genetic, and hormonal activity guide the differentiation of the sexes (Figure 5-6).

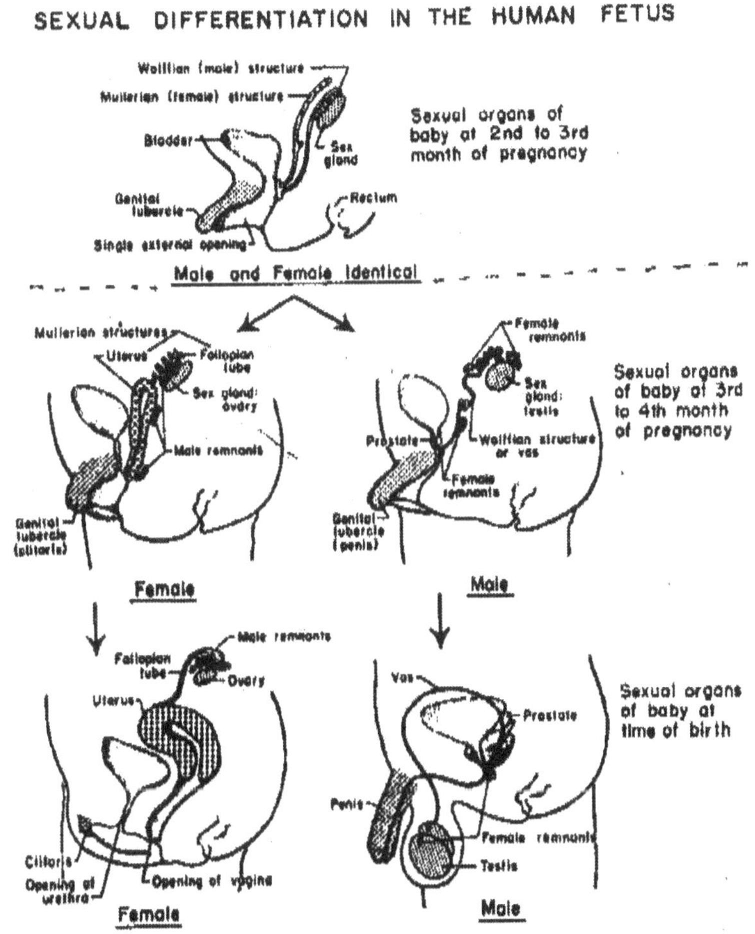

Figure 5-6 The sequence of events in development of a fetus that leads to male and female sexual characteristics under normal circumstances (from Money, p.41, Fig 3.1)

David Crew states the process very succinctly:

An embryo starts out having a mass of primordial (original) sexual tissue. Genetic signals determine whether that tissue develops into male or female gonads (ovary or testes). Subsequent hormonal triggers that act in the embryo control the sex of the genitalia. The testes of the genetic male produce significant concentration of androgen, which induce the formation of the vas deferens, a penis and a scrotum. In the absence of androgen, the embryo acquires female sexual organs; a uterus, a clitoris and vaginal labia. Accumulating evidence from animal experiments suggests that many components of adult sexuality—not just the structure of the sexual organs—depend on the hormonal environment during fetal development.[7]

All of these factors act with and respond to the varying conditions of the tissue environment of the fetus. Normal sexual differentiation depends on the nature of the chromosomal and hormonal signals and on the readiness of the developing tissues to respond to those signals. The readiness of the tissue is, in turn, a consequence of previous developmental events.

These previous developmental events, as we shall see, include the health habits, and diet of the mother.

Developmental Noise

Lewontin identifies the remaining and third source of variation in fetal development as developmental noise. Developmental noise is the consequence of chance events during development. This term does not refer to external environmental changes, but rather to the unscheduled happenings that disturb the critical developmental order of chromosomal and hormonal growth patterns just described.[8] Indeed, the physical and mental differences that are apparent at birth may not be the result of genetic differences, but rather a consequence of this so-called developmental noise. For example, small, accidental alterations in the growth pattern of nerve connections in the fetal brain may produce considerable differences in the mental functioning of the infant. Such differences may affect the individual's level of general intelligence, or perhaps his or her mathematical or verbal abilities. This phenomenon may explain why many people are able to play a musical instrument but only a few are virtuosos. To the extent that diet, exercise and psychological health can affect ordered growth, parents have some control over developmental noise. Let us consider brain development, which is directly and indirectly related to sexuality (a concept which is explored in Chapter 8), to see how developmental noise works.

By the end of the seventh week of pregnancy, perhaps before the pregnancy is even known or verified, more than 100,000 new nerve cells are being created in the brain every minute! Lewontin states that:

> Interconnections among millions of neurons in the brain that arise during the development of the embryo cannot possibly be specified

by genotype, even in a fixed environment. Developmental noise must play a role in the growth of the brain, perhaps a considerable one.[9]

In other words, if the environment of the womb were to be totally stable at all times, genes alone could not explain the millions of nerve interconnections in the brain. An example of how developmental noise is involved is demonstrated in the next paragraph.

The most serious nervous system defects can arise at the end of the first month of pregnancy, before a woman knows she is pregnant. The neural tube, later to become the brain and spinal cord, may fail to close completely, interfering with normal brain development. A study of 347 women who gave birth to babies with neural tube defects and 2,829 women whose babies were born without defects was conducted by Mulinare and his colleagues at the Center for Disease Control.[10] These researchers found that the risk of having infants with neural tube defects was 60 percent less in those women who reported taking vitamin supplements for at least three months before conception and during the first three months of pregnancy.[11] As we shall learn in a later chapter, recent studies have shown that brain development is clearly of extreme importance to sexual development. Moreover, a recent American Medical Association study of 22,000 women confirmed that the risk of disability in infants was lessened with vitamin intake.

What an incentive for prenatal care and education! (The reader should note however, that caution should be exercised, and expert advice sought by individual mothers, as vitamin overdoses can also cause birth defects. In this instance, more is not necessarily better.)

Thus a pregnant woman's diet, rest patterns, drug or alcohol intake, and level of exercise all play a role in providing an environment that either promotes or suppresses normal development of the child in the womb. In other words, all of these personal habits can influence the amount of developmental noise to which the fetus is subjected.

Even the use of hot tubs, at least in the first six weeks of pregnancy, is a documented cause of brain defects. Indeed, clinicians at the Boston University Medical School advise that oral and written notice about this practice be provided to women who are pregnant and to those considering pregnancy. Another example of the effect of the mother's health on her developing fetus is found in studies revealing the presence of lead in the umbilical cords of neonates whose mothers had higher-than-normal lead levels in their bodies.

The World Resources Institute found even a low level of hormone-disrupting chemicals were a cause of concern for couple's infertility. The University of Iowa found women working on farms from two to twenty times as likely to experience infertility. Seventy chemicals are known to be hormone-disrupters liable to change the endocrine system and cause neural birth defects. A study has found that the quality of semen is significantly poorer in men from rural mid-Missouri than in males from urban areas and its authors believe agricultural chemicals might explain the difference.[12] Facts such as these should be a part of everyone's general knowledge so that the increasing number of birth defects of moderate physical or mental impairment may be sharply decreased and hopefully eliminated.

Modern living has brought another influence.

Joseph Beasley, author of *The Betrayal of Health*, reminds us that the human embryo is extremely sensitive to the toxic substances in the environment, especially during the early stages when vital organs are forming. In fact, Beasley states: "Concern about the danger of environmental agents now extends back to the reproductive cells prior to conception." He attributes environmentally defective genes to the rapid rise in physical and mental disabilities in the last 25 years—an estimated 7 percent of all newborns now suffer some defect.[13]

In summary then, the three critical factors that influence sexual development are genes, hormones, and the physical and psychological environment of the womb. Present studies are attempting to target the precise timing and interaction of these factors. Moreover, environment is now known to be influenced by developmental noise, which in part is controlled by the environment and the personal habits of the mother. In turn, the personal habits of the mother can be influenced by the attitudes and personal habits of the father. Thus, pregnancy is not a *woman thing* but rather is—or should be—the concern of both parents.

It is also important to distinguish between gender determination and sex differentiation. Genetic sex determination is a matter normally settled at the beginning of development by the union of chromosomes. Sex differentiation goes on until maturity and is not always the expected expression of the genetic sex. If development proceeds normally, a boy develops testes and a girl develops ovaries. All of the secondary sex characteristics—such as size, body form, metabolism, and skeletal differences—are influenced by the sex hormones secreted by the ovaries and testes. It does not always follow that because chromosomes are of a certain type, the secondary sex characteristics will be similar. The genetic constitution of the parents may be immaterial in some cases. The gonads (ovaries and testes) release substances called sex hormones and it is these substances not the sex chromosomes which influence the development of accessory sexual organs.[14]

Such a complex interaction of genes and hormones with the critical timing which is important to the development and reception of this interaction may offer an explanation of why, during adolescence and into young adulthood, many individuals struggle with their sexual identity as their sexual organs are maturing. Often, young males struggle with fears of homosexuality at this time. Same sex activity and sexual abuse often occur. Their lack of knowledge and understanding of their sexual development adds greatly to their fears and experimentation. Teenage girls experience the same fears that very often are not brought to consciousness and therefore seldom resolved.

With this briefest of outlines, the reader will be able to see that the physical origins of our sexual identity can vary widely and can profoundly affect the degree to which our individual sexuality is developed. Moreover, these variations can be the direct result of biological occurrences in the womb whose influence extends not only to the creation of the infant, but also to one's development throughout one's lifetime.

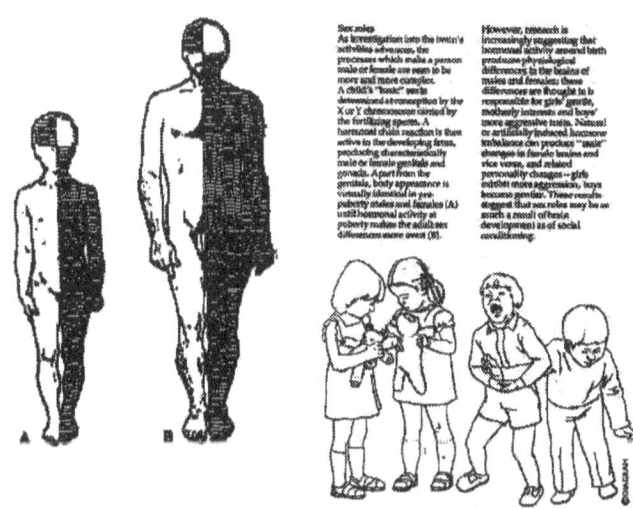

Figure 5-7 Sex and Sexuality Development from The Brain—A User's Manual, 1982, pp. 222-223

Ashley Montagu in his book *Prenatal Influences* is most emphatic on this point.

> It is during these nine prenatal months that the individual's foundations are well and truly laid—or not. To an extent rather more profound than we had hitherto suspected, the individual's prenatal past influences his postnatal future.... The prenatal past is, in fact, critically important, for upon the manner in which the individual's development proceeds within these nine months, the whole of his future will depend.[15]

By learning about the biological pattern of sexual development, parents (or prospective parents) can become more effective in helping their children learn about sexuality and gender in a comfortable non-threatening way.

In brief…

❖ Sexual identity begins in the womb.

❖ Sexual identity can be influenced—and indeed, changed—by the unique interaction of genes, hormones, and "developmental noise."

❖ In the womb, fetus tissue receptivity is necessary for hormones to promote normal development. The receptivity of the tissue is influenced by the attitudes and behavior of the mother, which are, in turn, influenced by the nurturing and receptive attitude of the father.

❖ Brain development, vital to sexual development, is vulnerable during the early weeks of pregnancy and can be influenced by healthy diet and vitamin supplements.

❖ The secondary sex characteristics of an adult may differ from the genetically determined sex of the infant.

Chapter 5—Endnotes

[1] Lewontin, Richard, *Human Diversity*, Scientific American Library, W.H. Freeman & Co., New York, NY, 1982

[2] Noble, Elizabeth, *Primal Connections*, Simon & Schuster, New York, NY, 1993

[3] Lewontin, op cit

[4] Ibid

[5] Moore, Keith L., *The Developing Human, Clinically Oriented Embryology*, Saunders Publishing Co., New York, NY 4th edition, 1988

[6] Lewontin, op cit p.125

[7] Crews, David, "Animal Sexuality", *Scientific American*, January 1994, pp. 109-114

[8] Lewontin, op cit p.97

[9] Ibid

[10] Mulinare, Dr. Joseph, "Readers Digest" April 1989, p.124—"Prevention Magazine" March 1990, pp127-128

[11] American Medical Association Study, "Wellness Today", *Special Supplement to Health and Healing*, April 1992

[12] University of Minnesota, Los Angeles Medical Center, University of California at Davis, Mount Sinai School of Medicine, AP Release *Daily Gazette*, 11/11/02

[13] Beasley, Joseph D. *The Betrayal of Health*, Times Book (Random House Incorporated) New York, 1991

[14] Michaelmore, Susan, *Sexual Reproduction*, Eyre & Soituswode, Ltd, (England) 1964. The American Museum of Natural History by the Natural Free Press, New York, NY

[15] Montagu, Ashley, M. D., *Prenatal Influences*, Charles C. Thomas, Springfield, Ill., 1962

Chapter 6

The Empathy Belly

Pre-anxiety can exist in fetal life without necessarily any psychic content...physical recording without conscious registration of experience within the fetal cortex...appears highly probable.

Ashley Montagu, M.D.[1]

Another consequence of the historical nature of organisms is that the way an organism reacts to a particular environment at a particular stage of life history depends on the environments of the past, which are somehow recorded in the organism's physiology and anatomy. In human beings, much information about past environment is stored in the immune system.

Richard Lewontin[2]

What a child feels and perceives begins shaping his attitudes and expectations about himself. Whether he ultimately sees himself, and hence acts, as a happy or sad, aggressive or meek, secure or anxiety-ridden person, depends, in part, on the message he gets about himself in the womb.

Thomas Verny, M.D.[3]

A child's response to his/her mother's feelings while growing in the womb is amazingly sensitive and as Verny points out, can literally shape the evaluation of self. Empathy Belly, a term borrowed from LaMaze childbirth preparation classes, seems an apt phrase to introduce the inherent connectedness of mother and embryo. It expresses well the influence of a mother's attitude on the unfolding of her infant's individuality and developing sexuality—the infant's beginning evaluation of self. Such connectedness is nature's way of helping us to nurture life from conception to death.

Development Of Self Esteem

The initial attitude to be considered is how the mother feels about herself. Does she hold herself in high esteem? What exactly is self-esteem?

The State of California deemed self-esteem to be so important that it authorized a survey and study of the subject. In 1990, *the California Task Force* gave its final report on the promotion of self-esteem and personal and social responsibility. The Task Force adopted the following as its official definition of self-esteem: "appreciating my own worth and importance and having the character to be accountable for myself and to act responsibly toward others." A very comprehensive definition!

Let us consider for a moment the first portion of that definition, "appreciating our own worth." True self-worth is not an instant recognition process but a life-long struggle to learn and maintain our true identity. True self-worth is not identical with self-esteem. A true evaluation of one's worth is principally developed from within although influenced by interaction with others. So many of us never truly appreciate our own dignity, allowing the opinion and approval of others to form our sense of worth. Maturity includes the ability to feel good about yourself without someone else's approval.

If we look only to others for approval and self-affirmation, the fear of not being loved can keep us from admitting that we are not perfect. In order to feel good about ourselves, we may often deny our imperfections, subsequently developing defenses to guard against anyone else discovering them. In so doing, we are not so much appreciating our own worth, but some myth or fabrication of self-worth that is based on others perceptions—self-worth once removed, as it were!

Psychiatrist and author, Dr. Scott Peck's distinction between self-esteem—the goal of the California study—and self-love (self-worth) is very enlightening in this regard.[4] Self-esteem, he believes, is a somewhat arguable goal, as the guarding of it, in fear of not being loved, may lead the person away from self-knowledge.

Self-knowledge is the basis of true self-love—of appreciating one's own worth. It is true self-love rather than self-esteem (which the dictionary defines as pride in one's self) that allows us to love others. Psychology tells us that we cannot love others unless we first love ourselves. Most of us believe that self-love begins at birth, or later. Not so. For each of us, self-love and the ability to love others begins in the womb. The formation of our self-image begins with the primitive impressions that we, as fetuses, derive from the womb environment—ideally, an accepting womb environment. These impressions, loving or not, are then confirmed or revised according to experiences outside the womb, depending on the degree to which an infant senses or receives acceptance or rejection during development. These early impressions, then have an impact on the formation of each individual personality, and on the capacity of that individual to give or receive love.

Do you find this hard to believe? There is perhaps no better example for demonstrating this principle than Verny provides in his book, *The Secret Life of the Unborn*.[5] In it, Verny recounts the experience of his colleague, Dr. Peter Fedor-Freybergh, in relation to Kristina, a healthy infant who was born after a seemingly uneventful pregnancy. After birth, Kristina, unlike other healthy babies, refused to nurse at her mother's breast. However, when fed by bottle in the nursery, she drank hungrily. Believing that something was amiss, Fedor-Freybergh arranged for another lactating mother to breastfeed the child. There was no hesitancy; Kristina sucked vigorously. Intrigued, the doctor questioned Kristina's mother about any prior illness or any experience that might give meaning to Kristina's behavior. Finally, he asked, "Well, did you want to get pregnant then?" The woman looked up and said, "No, I didn't. I wanted an abortion. My husband wanted the child. That's why I had her." Apparently, Kristina had sensed rejection from the womb, and had refused to bond with her mother. What a strong statement for a four-day-old child! What a powerful example of the capacity of the infant in the womb!

The Womb As A Medium For Experience

Specifically, what are some of the messages—both physical and emotional—that infants receive in their individual worlds in the womb, and how do they react? The intrauterine environment is not as protective as we once believed. Many toxins in the workplace have been shown to cause birth defects as do environmental pollutants. As mentioned before, these substances can also injure the sperm and egg prior to conception or they can penetrate the placental barrier and damage the embryo or fetus, contributing to disabilities after birth.

Chemical Stimulation

A growing human being begins to learn of the world and other-than-self experiences as development progresses in the noisy atmosphere of the womb, where the fetus is protected to some extent by floating in the surrounding amniotic sac. In 24 days the fetus is encased is what Sara Stein calls a "space suit"[6] bringing from the mother her oxygen, her food and dumping into the mother's its waste. Accordingly, it is easy to comprehend how the mother's daily habits and the quality of her environment govern the amount of oxygen the baby receives. (Figure 6-1)

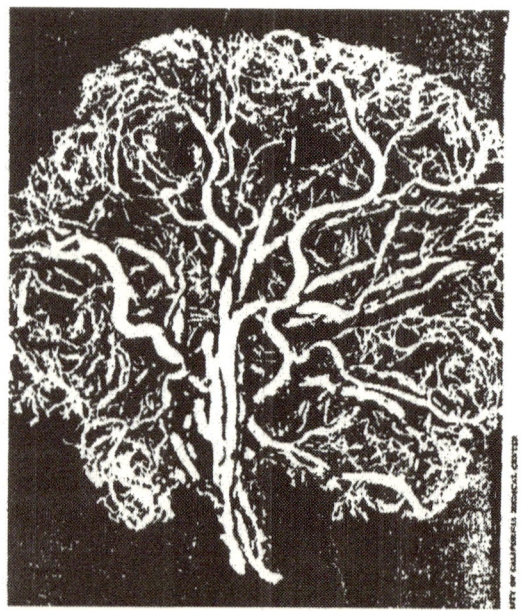

Figure 6-1 The tree of life for the baby is this growth of vessels in the placenta. All supplies of food and oxygen come to the baby through these vessels, and all the wastes are removed through them. The vessels here are plainly visible because they have been stripped of the surrounding tissues of the placenta in a special corrosion process (from Flanagan, Geraldine Lux, *The First Nine Months of Life*, Simon & Schuster, 2nd Edition, New York, NY. 1982 p. 90)

To emphasize the close union of fetus and mother consider that the placenta helps the mother to cooperate with her developing pregnancy. It contains hormones which keep the womb relaxed and enrich its lining. It looks ahead to future needs and secrets hormones to grow the milk glands in the mother's breast. When it comes time for the baby to be born, hormones from the placenta loosen the mother's hip joints so the baby can slide through. Nature really thinks of everything!

However, to return to the habits of the mother—if she is a smoker, the baby will be dramatically affected by this practice, both physically and emotionally. Investigations conducted as early as 1935 have demonstrated that, eight or ten minutes after the mother finishes her cigarette, the baby's heartbeat increases 39 beats per minute. In fact a 1970 review of this study found that a baby's heartbeat increases when the mother merely thinks about smoking. Apparently, the mother produces a chemical reaction in her body in anticipation of smoking, which then crosses the placental barrier and stimulates the fetal heart.

Verny notes that:

> ...the drop in the oxygen supply (smoking lowers the oxygen con-
> tent of the maternal blood passing through the placenta), is physio-
> logically harmful to him [the fetus], but possibly even more harmful
> are the psychological effects of maternal smoking. It thrusts him into
> a chronic state of uncertainty and fear. He never knows when that
> unpleasant physical sensation will reoccur, or how painful it will be
> when it does, only that it will reoccur. And that's the kind of situa-
> tion which may predispose [an individual] toward a deep-seated,
> conditioned anxiety.[7]

Likewise, the fetus' reaction to drugs (prescribed or otherwise) taken by the mother is profound. Although the mother's body has the ability to break down an adult dose and transform it for use in her body, fetuses do not have this capacity, and so their development may be deeply affected by the introduction of even small amounts of such toxic substances. Cocaine, during early pregnancy, can cause miscarriage. In later stages, it can cause death or irreversible brain damage. Consider, too, that the effect of nicotine and other drugs is intergenerational. The embryo's developing ovary contains all the eggs for the next generation when still in the uterus of the mother; that means that diet and other factors in the life of the pregnant woman could have a direct impact not only on her children but on the grandchildren who will be produced from the egg cells forming in her embry-onic daughter. Thus the effects on environment can potentially be transmitted across generations.[8]

It is true that a recent study by the Center for Disease Control noted a drop in the rate of smoking by pregnant women to just over 12% (a half-million moth-ers). However, the rate of white teen-agers who smoke rose to 30%, a fact that doesn't bode well for future generations. This study showed various rates for the different ethnic groups with Chinese women rating the lowest at 0.5 percent.

In this information age, one would think new mothers would understand alcohol affects their fetus. Unfortunately, fetal alcohol syndrome is one of the three leading causes of birth defects according to the New York Department of Health and the Center for Disease Control. Maternal drinking is increasing across the nation. In 1998 in Buffalo, the rate of babies born with fetal alcohol syndrome was three times the national average. Three of every 1000 babies were diagnosed with FAS according to the NYS Department of Health and the Center for Disease Control. One in 20 women drink during pregnancy.

Physical and mental disabilities have increased over the last twenty-five years. At present, an estimated 7% of all newborns suffer some defect.[9]

Auditory Stimulation

The baby in the womb also learns of its world through sound. Again, smoking interferes with development. Newborns, born of mothers who smoked during pregnancy, tested at birth and later (ages 6-11), revealed abnormalities in auditory processing at both stages. Compared with children of mothers who had not smoked during pregnancy, these children demonstrated that they had difficulty distinguishing words. Auditory capacity develops as early as twenty-eight weeks after conception, and is facilitated by the amniotic sac being a more effective sound conductor than air. Besides the sounds of the mother's body—her heartbeat, the blood flowing through arteries and veins, and the rumblings of the digestive tract (proven through recordings)—the infant hears outside sounds as diverse as washing machines and concert music. In support of this theory, Verny cites the experience of a music conductor who was puzzled by his apparent foreknowledge of certain movements of symphonic music, a "knowledge" that allowed him to conduct unfamiliar scores of the music without previous rehearsal. He finally discovered that his mother, a cellist, had practiced that same music over and over while she was carrying him in her womb![10]

The infant also becomes familiar with certain voices while in the womb, especially that of the mother. Indeed, her patterns of speech, heard prenatally, are said to affect the child's early language development. Our speech patterns are as unique as our fingerprints. We copy our speech patterns from our mother and this learning begins in the womb. Infants have even been noted to synchronize their body rhythms with their mother's speech! What good reasons for Mom and Dad to talk to their baby in the womb! At birth, the baby recognizes these familiar voices and is reassured by the sound after the long birth journey into a strange world. In fact, the familiar melody of a lullaby that has been sung to an infant while in the womb will usually be effective in quieting that same baby after birth.

In his clinic outside of Paris, Dr. Odent, author and educator encourages singing by the prospective parents who attend his workshops.[11] Singing and socializing serves the dual purpose of helping mothers and their unborn babies feel happy while information about childbearing can be exchanged informally. Noble calls this contact with the baby in utero "prenatal enrichment."[12]

Light Stimulation

Unborn babies within the womb can distinguish light from the outside world—even if their mother is merely sunbathing. If a light is shone directly on the mother's stomach, the child will turn its head away. If the baby is startled enough, this stimulus will increase its heart rate dramatically.

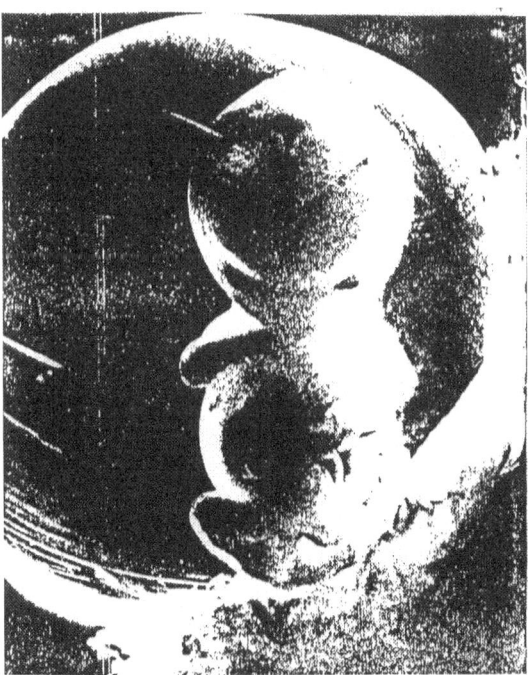

Figure 6-2 7-week-old human fetus is about an inch long. Eyes and limbs are visible, and the emerging brain is apparent. Stimulation is needed to complete development, a process that for many neural systems continues into neonatal life (Carla J. Schatz, *The Developing Brain* from Scientific American 9/92, p. 60)

Stress

Likewise, the baby's level of in utero activity increases dramatically when the mother is upset. Consider that every time a mother breathes, she varies the intrauterine pressure for her child. Given the fact that a person's emotional state affects his or her breathing pattern, it becomes clear how messages of acceptance and love can be conveyed to the infant in the womb and a welcoming environment provided or conversely, how emotional upheaval can have an unsettling, negative effect on the infant.

The unconditional acceptance and love of the mother during pregnancy gives the unborn child a sense of being loved and loveable. You might ask, how do we know this? If one accepts the premise that, at conception, all three systems: physical, psychological and spiritual come to bear on that child's development, it seems logical.

However, in addition to logic, there have been numerous reports of the effects of stress on the unborn child. One consistent finding among them is that, rather than external stress, it is the accepting or rejecting attitude of the mother (both unconscious and conscious) that most deeply affects the emotional and physical health of the child.

Dr. Antonio Ferreira, in his study of *Emotional Factors in Prenatal Development*, cites three distinct categories in which the emotional state of the mother is reflected in reproductive events:

1. Infertility—a number of cases have been reported successfully treated by psychotherapy.

2. Adoption followed by a woman's unexpected pregnancy indicates an impact on the reproductive system; a wish to have (or not to have) a baby.

3. Habitual spontaneous abortion occurred frequently in women with emotional conflicts with regard to having a family. Psychotherapy has also proven successful with a number of these individuals.

It is fair to say that not all such events are emotionally triggered in all women, but, indications are of sufficient number to underscore science's findings that a mother's negative attitude towards pregnancy may be, by different means, conveyed to the fetus and reflected in complications of pregnancy or in the child's early deviant behavior.[13]

When one takes into account the amazing physical changes taking place in the womb—which are more numerous than at any other time in a child's development—it is easy to believe that the child would benefit from the knowledge that it is loved and wanted. Reassured in this way, the unborn infant's energy can be directed to the developmental events at hand, rather than diverted to deal with vague, unsettling perceptions of rejection.

As stated in the previous chapter, exposure to excessive or insufficient amounts of maternal hormones can produce biologically induced sexual changes in an unborn child. Likewise, excessive and rapid changes in the neurohormonal system of the mother, usually triggered by the mother's fears, anger, or rejection can produce similar effects on a child's neurological circuitry.

One may ask, if there is no connection between the mother's nervous system and that of the fetus, and there is no anatomical connection, how can the mother's emotional states, originating in the nervous system, act on the fetus? Dr. Ashley Montagu, in *Prenatal Influences* clarifies this pathway.

> The mother's emotional states are able to affect the fetus because they operate not within the nervous system alone, but through the nervous system in interaction with the endocrine glandular system…. This is the neurohormonal system. The endocrine secretions of the mother and those of the fetus together form a common endocrine pool, and it is this that forms the neurohormonal bond between them. The endocrine system of the mother and fetus complement each other. There is reciprocal transmission of hormones between mother and fetus across the placenta.
>
> Stimuli, then impinging upon the mother and originating changes in the grey matter of her brain can indirectly produce significant changes in the mother's neurohormonal system, which can, in turn, more or less directly affect the development of the fetus.[14]

Dependency of the embryo in utero on the emotional and physical state of the mother is an idea that is becoming more understandable as we recognize the effect of stress on our bodies. Indeed, one researcher[15] has gone so far as to suggest that an individual's homosexual orientation may correlate with state of the mother's hormones during pregnancy, although this notion is not widely accepted. In any case, it seems valid to assert that unconditional love allows normal neurological development by providing a hospitable womb. This concept becomes more believable as we learn more of the effect of stress on our own bodies and the connection of emotional support with our physical health.

Verny (cited previously) compares the progress of the child to a computer that is continually being programmed. As the brain matures, unborn children move from simple neural receptors to the ability to make more connections. At three months in utero they may only be able to respond on a primitive level to maternal feelings of ambivalence and coolness. Researchers have even elicited reflexes as early as the seventh or eighth week of development when the emerging brain is apparent.

Dr. Dominick Pupura reports in recent neurological studies that the start of awareness is pinpointed between the 28th and 32nd week of gestation[16] At this point, the brain's neural circuitry is believed to be as developed as that of a newborn infant. By the end of gestation, the infant is able to respond with great accuracy to maternal feelings.

Dr. M.M.I. Liley,[17] believes that infants, in utero, trigger the physical changes in the mother's body that nourish them. The placenta, considered an organ of the infant, produces many hormones necessary to maintain pregnancy. By determining the endocrine balance during gestation, unborn infants actively participate and exert some control over their survival.

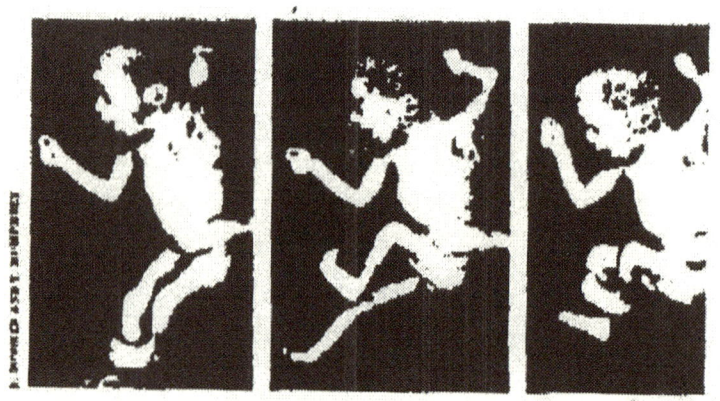

Figure 6-3 The vigorous personality of this baby is apparent in these motion picture films taken in the sixth month (from Flanagan, p.107)

During both physical and emotional maternal stress periods, the unborn child becomes emotionally volatile because his or her body machinery has been significantly altered by an excess flow of maternal neurohormones. The child will continue to grow and develop after birth, but this development will be governed, in part, by prenatal experiences. Sontag named this phenomenon somatopsychics.[18] He defined it as the way "basic physiological processes affect the personality structure, perception and performance of the individual." (This phenomenon is not to be confused with a psychosomatic condition in which personality predisposes the body toward such illnesses as ulcers or hypertension.)

Sensations associated with anxiety, depression, and excitement start in the hypothalamus, located at the base of the brain, but the specific physical changes that such emotions produce are created by the two centers it controls: the endocrine system and the autonomic nervous system.

The autonomic system, as the word implies, is independent of conscious control; it affects the digestive organs, heart, and other organs that work without direction from the conscious mind. When working normally, the body has a sense of well-being. When stress and danger prevail, the autonomic nervous system is activated. (When we are excited, we can influence these two systems by deep breathing. In light of this, industry now recommends meditation and relaxation to employees as a means of improving their performance and emotional health.)

When a pregnant woman becomes frightened, the hypothalamus "orders" the autonomic nervous system to respond by increasing the heart rate, dilating the pupils, making the palms sweat, and increasing the blood pressure. Collectively, these changes signal the body to step up neurohormonal production (i.e., adrenaline and noradrenaline). As these substances enter the blood, they affect the mother's glands and cross into the placenta, altering the child's body processes as well. Just at what point the fetal brain is most vulnerable to these kinds of changes is not known. It is theorized that the child's hypothalamus can be set too high or too low by the mother's neurohormonal activity. Such dysfunction in the mother can possibly affect the subsequent function of the endocrine system and nervous system of the child.[19]

Studies of pregnant women during World War I explored the effects of stress on the children born during this troubled time. Sontag reports on one study which focused on those pregnant women whose husbands were in battle, and a second study on women who gave birth during the famine caused by a war food embargo.[20]

The results of the second study—of offspring born during the war famine of 1944 in Holland—revealed that severe overweight problems were common in these children. Suffering severe hunger during the first four months of gestation was thought to have the greatest effect on subsequent weight disorders. From this research, it was concluded that nutritional deprivation during that period affected the setting of the "appestat"—that area of the hypothalamus that regulates food intake and growth.

Sontag revealed that children who were in utero when their fathers died in battle were more likely to develop psychiatric disorders than those children whose fathers died shortly after the children were born. Again, researchers concluded that the hypothalamus had been adversely affected by the maternal distress.

Of course, these were cases of extreme distress, but one cannot help recalling the old wives' tale of fear and anxiety making its mark on the infant. Perhaps it was an intuitive guess at what science is now discovering—that the womb environment is affected by maternal feelings and the mother's daily habits. As the mother is stimulated, whether in love or anger, she passes it along to her baby and the infant reacts. It is a form of learning that stays with the baby. Could a disturbance of the hypothalamus during pregnancy be a contributing factor to the fact that 2% to 5% of adolescent women suffer from anorexia and bulimia? It would be interesting to find out.

There are also potential benefits to be derived from the common emotions experienced by the mother during pregnancy provided these emotions are not extreme in either duration or intensity. Schwartz, who believes that ego formation begins in the womb maintains that: "anxiety—a common maternal emotion...disturbs his [the fetus] sense of oneness with his surroundings and makes him aware of his own separateness and distinctness. It also pushes him into action. Being excited...he kicks, he squirms, devising ways to get out—in short, he starts erecting a set of primitive defense mechanisms."[21]

Anxiety of the mother, it appears, has a two-fold effect. The *degree* of anxiety would seem to be a controlling factor.

Potentially, the second most powerful influence producing stress perceived within the womb environment is the stability of the parents' relationship, whether in or out of wedlock. Fathers can play an important part here. A woman's relationship with her partner or spouse should be a happy, affirming one. Fathers need to recognize that a mother's need for nurturance and support increases before and after the birth of their child. Based on studies of more than 1,300 children and their families, Dr. Dennis Stott estimates that a woman who is locked in a stormy marriage has a 237 percent greater risk of bearing a psychologically or physically damaged child than does a woman who is in a stable, nurturing relationship. Furthermore, the offspring of those women in a troubled marriage, even at five years of age continue to be plagued by problems of timidity and emotional dependence on the mother.[22]

These studies do not mean, however, that a strong mother-child bond cannot overcome very traumatic shocks.

Verny states this concept so well:

> There are no one-to-one correlations in human psychology. Because a child is the product of an unhappy marriage or the baby of a cool, ambivalent or even catastrophic mother does not necessarily mean he will develop an adult case of mental illness. Nothing about the mind is that neat. But the womb is the child's first world. How he experiences it—as friendly or hostile—does create personality and character predispositions. The womb, in a very real sense, establishes a child's expectations. If it has been a warm, loving environment, the child is likely to expect the outside world to be the same. This produces a predisposition toward trust, openness, extroversion and self-

confidence. The world will be his oyster, just as the womb has been. If that environment has been hostile, the child will anticipate that his new world will be equally uninviting. He will be predisposed toward suspiciousness, distrust and introversion. Relating to others will be hard, and so will self assertion. Life will be more difficult for him than [for] a child who had a good womb experience.[23]

We began this chapter with a discussion about self-love/worth. A firm foundation for the development of self-love is afforded those children fortunate enough to have the good womb experience Verny describes. This self-love, in turn, will provide the underpinnings for their ability to love others. The emotional well-being of the child is secured by the psychological development and maturity of both parents. The inter-connectedness of us all is startling, especially at the time of pregnancy (Figure 6-4).

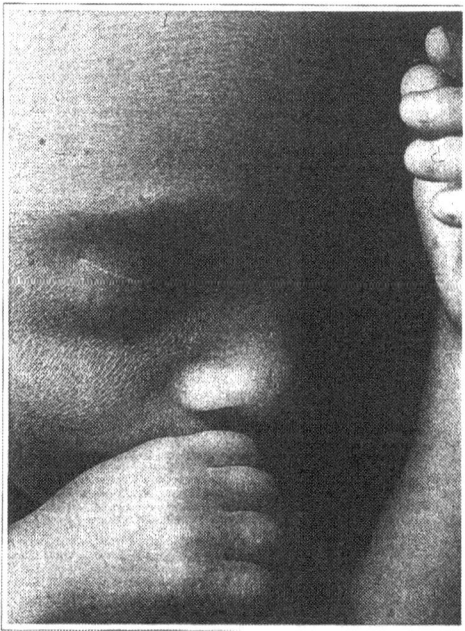

Figure 6-4 A fetus from the fifth month of pregnancy, peacefully sucking its thumb, The gesture with the left hand is not reflexive, but changes in accordance with the embryo's brain waves. Most features are completely formed, as seen in the presence of the right eyebrow and the fingernail on the left hand. The remaining four months will be mostly steady enlargement. (from David Bodanis, The Body Book: A Fantastic Voyage to the World Within)

Parents, however, have many pressures with which to contend. The societal climate today makes even a welcomed pregnancy more difficult in many ways. Having a baby is often perceived as an obstacle for women to succeed in a man's world, or an impingement on the freedom of a woman. In a male-dominated society, growing a baby is the least masculine act a woman can possibly perform. Nor does the woman normally get paid for it, which is a powerful message in a society that values money so highly. Even in the context of a normal, welcomed pregnancy, occasional fears, regrets, and feelings of ambivalence arise to over-shadow the joy and excitement of creating new life. Added to these mixed feelings are new concerns related to recent discoveries about the effects of hormones, genes, medications, drugs, and alcohol. All parents wonder and worry about whether their baby will be healthy and perfect, at the same time wrestling with the imminent burdens of soaring medical costs, loss of wages, and possible loss of career (See Table 6-A, end of Chapter for a list of such feelings).

Making a baby brings into question the parents' marriage, their relationship to their own parents and their personal beliefs about the world the newborn child will enter. These doubts, fears, and conflicts are not always conscious, and in some part may be the natural result of the tremendous physical and emotional changes occurring in the mother.

Pediatrician Dr. Niles Newton's book, *The Family Book on Child Care*,[24] was my bible during my own childbearing years, and it is still a reliable guide. (Childbearing has been the same since history began; it is just that we are becoming more aware of all it entails!) Newton gives excellent advice on the mixed feelings of motherhood. There is much to learn about the feelings and relationship changes for parents, especially in the first trimester of pregnancy, and those changes continue during the entire pregnancy and after the birth of the child. Schwartz outlines these changes well in her book, *The World of the Unborn*, quoted previously. Most important to remember is that the quality of the relationship between husband and wife can affect the development of the child in the womb. As we shall see in subsequent chapters, it is also a primary factor in the formation of the child's sexuality after birth.

Do messages in the womb have a bearing on the development of adult sexuality? If self-love and our self-image are formed, however primitively, in the womb, then it follows that our adult sexuality will reflect that image. Indeed, this premise is borne out by a study conducted by Verny of a number of patients who had expressed a belief that there was a correlation between their subjective womb feelings and their adult sexual behavior. Verny reported,

> People who recalled being terrified in utero were markedly more
> unsure of themselves sexually and also prone to sexual problems,

while those who remembered the womb as a good and peaceful place were sexually better adjusted.[25]

Elizabeth Noble claims that those who sense rejection in the womb, often seek what they missed in later sexual behavior.

> Epilepsy, tics, stuttering and sex are ways that people discharge tension. What many people want out of sex is actually touch rather than sex. They desire the warmth, protection, love, closeness and reassurance that touch brings and the price they are willing to pay is [genital] sex.[26]

Rejection of pregnancy and unhappy marriages do occur, however, all too frequently. So, what can be done to protect the unborn? What affects the child's development is not occasional personal stress, but that which is long-term, continuous and a problem that has no foreseeable resolution.

Booth Maternity Center in Philadelphia, Pennsylvania has pioneered a partial solution: a counseling program whereby parent(s)-to-be not only receive necessary medical attention and education, but also are counseled to cope with the conflicting emotional problems that unhappy conditions provoke. During the question-and-answer period that followed a talk I gave at our local YWCA, one woman, encouraged by my description of the services at Booth, related how her sister had benefited by Booth's program. Her sister had rejected her pregnancy strongly at the beginning. She was able to change her attitudes during the course of the counseling until, at the time of birth, she was free to accept her child with love. Such counseling should be made available nationwide as part of low-cost conventional obstetrical services.

To echo Newton's first rule for parents-to-be: "Learn the facts about pregnancy, childbirth and the care of the newborn." I would add another caveat to that advice. Do not wait to learn those facts until you are pregnant. Rather, the process of education should be an ongoing inquiry that is initiated early. The last chapter of this book details specific strategies for facilitating that educational process.

As we educate ourselves, we begin the cyclical process of educating the next generation. We will pass on what we learn and believe—and more importantly, what we do—to our children in many unconscious ways. One of our first priorities as parents is to teach children good health habits and of course, to practice them. They should be taught how their bodies work so that they, in turn, can bring to parenthood an accepting environment—healthy in all areas of body, mind and spirit.

In brief...

❖ Self-love begins on a primitive level in the womb.

❖ Nurturing attitudes on the part of both parents are necessary for the development of self-love that, in turn, affects adult sexuality.

❖ The psychological and neurological development of the fetus is affected by hunger (diet), smoking, light, and sound, as well as the fears and anxieties of the parents.

❖ Strategies must be developed to ensure a hospitable womb for each child. This means the availability of quality prenatal care and early education on the formation and function of our bodies.

Table 6-A

Possible Emotions and Feelings During Pregnancy

FIRST 3 MONTHS (1-12 WEEKS)	SECOND 3 MONTHS (13-24 WEEKS)	THIRD 3 MONTHS (24-40 WEEKS)	POSTMARTUM REINTEGRATION
• Ambivalence and uncertainty, even when pregnancy is planned	• Increased dreams, fantasies; uncensored emotional reactions	• Ambivalence towards changing baby	• Need for mother-child bonding
• Joy, Pride in fertility	• Introspection	• Pride in full-blown pregnancy; reveling in role of life-giver (identification with divine aspects of motherhood, female myth goddess).	• Need for affection, reassurance, praise, security
• Fear of incompetence; fear of harming fetus	• Heightened awareness of unconscious processes	• Impatience with physical discomfort	• Celebratory period.
• Acceptance of pregnancy.	• Sense of excitement and reality in experiencing "quickening" of baby; awareness of irreversibility of events	• Need for affection and recognition of special state	• Emotional swings due to worries about competence in breastfeeding, mothering the baby, role as lover and partner.
• Vulnerability	• Free-floating anxiety	• Fear of death; Fear of letting go; fear of labor and delivery	• New sense of identity needs personal integration.
• Loss of control: natural process is talking over.	• Thoughts about one's own mother, transition from daughter to mother with accompanying conflicts and fears.	• Fears of separation from the baby.	• Need for social reintegration into community.
• Fear of dependency; concerns about trust	• Shift in dependency from mother to husband	• Anxiety about maternal capability.	
• Freedom in sex; heightened sexuality, no worry about contraception. Occasional fear of harming fetus during sex.		• Discomfort with increased fetal activity and size, sense of being invaded.	
• Moodiness; unpredictability; increased awe in relation to pregnant state; emotional sensitivity		• Insomnia; awkwardness.	
• Increased need for love and affection		• Nesting; excited preparation for baby's arrival, naming, fixing crib, etc.	

Chapter 6—Endnote

[1] Montagu Ashley, MD, *Prenatal Influences*, Charles C. Thomas, Springfield, Ill, 1962

[2] Lewontin, Richard, *Human Diversity*, Scientific American Library, Scientific American Books, W. H. Freeman & Co., New York, N. Y., 1982

[3] Verny, Thomas, M.D., with John Kelly, *The Secret Life of the Unborn*, Summit Books, Division of Simon & Schuster, New York, N.Y., 1981

[4] Peck, Scott, M.D., *Tape on Self-love vs. Self-esteem*, Simon & Schuster Audioworks, New York, N.Y., 1989

[5] Verny, op cit.

[6] Sara Stein, *The Body Book*, Workman Publishing, New York, 1992, P. 14

[7] Ibid, p. 21

[8] Ricklefs, Robert E., and Finch, Caleb E., *Aging, A Natural History*, Scientific American Library, W.N. Freeman, New York, N. Y., 1995

[9] Beasley, Joseph D. M.D., *The Betrayal of Health*, Times Book (Random House Incorporated)New York, 1991

[10] Verny, Ibid p.22

[11] Odent, Michael, *Primal Health: A Blueprint for Our Survival*, London Century, 1986

[12] Noble, Elizabeth, *Primal Connections*, Simon & Schuster, New York, N.Y., 1993

[13] Ferreira, Anthony, J., M.D., "Emotional Factors in Prenatal Environment", *Journal of Nervous and Mental Disease*, Vol. 141, No. 1, 1965

[14] Montagu, Dr. Ashley, *Prenatal Influences*, Charles C. Thomas, Springfield, Ill., 1962 p. 1993

[15] Hutchinson, Michael, *The Anatomy of Sex and Power, An Investigation of Mind-Body Politics*, Marrow Publishing Co., New York, N.Y., 1990

[16] Pupura, Dominick, M.D. *editor of "Brain Research"*, professor of Albert Einstein Medical College

[17] Liley, M.M.I., M.D., as cited by Scwartz, *The World of the Unborn*, Marek Publishers, New York, N.Y., 1980

[18] Sontag, Lester W., "War and the Fetal Maternal Relationship", *Marriage and Family Living* 6, pp. 1-5, 1944

[19] Verny, op cit

[20] Sontag, Lester W., "Implications of Fetal Behavior and Environment for Adult Personality", *Annals of New York Academy of Sciences*, pp.782-786, February 1966

[21] Schwartz, op cit

[22] Stott, Dennis, "Follow-up Study from Birth of the Effects of Prenatal Stress". *Developmental Medicine and Child Neurology*, vol. 15, pp 770-787, 1973

[23] Verny, op cit, p. 41

[24] Newton, Niles, M. D., *The Family Book of Child Care*, Harper & Brothers Publishers, New York, N. Y., 1957

[25] Verny, op cit, p.71

[26] Noble, op. cit.

Chapter 7

Our Invisible Being

It was you who created my inmost self, and put
me together in my mother's womb.
I thank you for the wonder of myself.

Psalm 139 (15-16)

Every person is linked to God from the moment of birth to the night of
his death by an invisible thread, a thread which is unique for each of us; a
thread which can never be broken, but a thread that can easily slip from
our grasp and elude us, despite searching. Our bodies are at the lowest
point of this thread which runs up through every sphere of heart and head
and spiritual attachment.

Irene Claremont de Castillejo, M.D[1]

The connection to the Divine is described by psychiatrist de Castellejo as a "thread that can never be broken but can easily slip from our grasp and elude us."[2] The thread de Castellejo refers to is unconditional love. Unconditional love at the beginning of life nourishes this spiritual capacity possessed by every human being. Such nourishment at this critical time provides a basis for future growth. Although spirit is truly limitless and indefinable, all of us can find examples of it in our daily lives as well as in the lives of famous people. Consider, for example, the courageous and generous spirit of Maximillian Kolbe who had been imprisoned in a German concentration camp and who offered his own life so that a father of a family might live; or the pluck of the little-known man who lifted a car off his chest in a Herculean effort to save his own life. Such happenings attest to the existence of the human spirit, the ability to transcend ourselves—to go beyond our own strength or knowledge in a given situation. In our modern world we often describe a person with spirit as enthusiastic. Some of us may realize such a description is derived from the Greek word enthorisiamos, meaning "in God."

For me, spirit may be defined as the breath of life or the spark of love from Divine Love that gives an individual the capacity to bring meaning to life and the motivation to act.

Jack Needleman, professor of philosophy at San Francisco State University, laments the inability of philosophers to answer such questions as; What is reality? Does God exist? Questions he terms "of the heart." He says these questions rise up because of something intrinsic in our nature.[3]

One aspect of this is the striving to participate in a reality greater than ourselves. It is a yearning, a hunger, a force we may recognize as love. This drive is as much, if not more, a part of our nature as the sexual physical desires which psychoanalysis and mainstream psychiatry have identified as parts of our essential nature. Our drive for understanding, for participation in a higher reality, shapes our psyche as much as anything else!

Elizabeth Noble, educator of birthing practices, strongly agrees. She says: "The purpose of your life is the same for all of us. Namely to get back in touch with your own divinity."[4]

This spiritual capacity or drive is present at conception and acts and reacts in the womb. Essentially, it is the ability of an individual to respond, an ability that can be wounded when the person is required to respond to indifference or hostility—the result of a lack of unconditional love. The intellect and emotions that are the psychological "fuel" for an individual's spiritual capacity have an impact on spiritual growth, either negatively or positively, depending on the specific instance. Out of our spiritual capacity develops what Freud called the superego and what is sometimes known as conscience. In addition, in past years, doctors have often documented the positive effect of faith on the healing of physical and mental illness but until recently the phenomenon has not been ascribed sufficient importance to warrant its universal acceptance.

However, recently Dr Sidney M. Jourard, professor of psychology and practicing psychotherapist, has actually proposed a method for measuring spirit called spirit titre, whereby spirit is conceptualized according to a numerical scale that ranges from zero to one-hundred, with the normal spirit titre being forty-five. Such descriptions as "his spirit is free" or "he is in high spirits" denote a mode of wellness. When the spirit titre falls below twenty or thirty units, the person is considered to be low-spirited and illness can occur. According to Jourard,

> The average person, behaves typically in ways that keeps his spirit titre considerably below the upper limit.... Wellness appears to ensue from such events as having one's individuality respected and acknowledged.... Being heard and touched by another who "cares" seems to reinforce identity, mobilize spirit and promote self healing.... Being the recipient of love appears to be a highly inspiring event. Previously dispirited people increased in zeal, muscle tone, integration of personality and resilience to illness once they were told they were loved by some significant other person.[5]

In attempting to pinpoint the unconditional stimuli that evoke faith, confidence, or an increase in spirit titre, Jourard concludes: "the assurance of a mother or a father mediated by cuddling, hugging or other symbols of protection, care or effort on one's own behalf—these may be the cues that inspire faith and surges of spirit."

The Spirit Of The Unborn

When a woman recognizes she is pregnant, much attention is (as it should be) directed to the physical health of the growing fetus and its mother. What is usually not considered is the emotional and spiritual health of both persons, although awareness is slowly growing. By spiritual, we are not referring to religious beliefs, but rather an innate vital principle that directs the individual, even in the womb, toward the integrity of personhood. The movement of the egg and sperm toward one another in perfect harmony is rooted in the living body of the parents and in their life experience. In less than one hour, as the sperm nucleus and the egg nucleus combine, instructed by genes, the traits of a new individual are decided—the color of the eyes, the tendency to be short or tall, the tendency for disease, and certain qualities of intelligence. But what gives the "breath of life" to the rapidly developing individuated cells formed by this process? I call it spirit—that thread of connection to the Divine.

The ideal spiritual environment in the womb is provided by a mother who genuinely desires and is ready to accept a child with all that acceptance demands of her and her husband.

As we all know, oxygen for the baby (the physical breath) is received from the mother via the placenta. This is why fresh air for the mother is so important during pregnancy. The baby is attached by a cord to the placenta, through which all life processes are performed. Even so, long before the infant's lungs and brain are ready to assume effective respiration, the baby begins practicing inhaling and exhaling movements. These practice sessions allow the amniotic fluid that envelops the baby to bathe the lining of the lungs, and is believed to be essential to the proper formation of the lung air sacs. How does the fetus know how to do this?

By the end of the second month, the baby forming in the womb is responding to touch, and thus can be said to be displaying the breath of life, or love, we call spirit. By the end of the twelfth week of gestation, the baby is not only responding, but is initiating activity and reflexes that are individual to him or her. As previously quoted, Dr. M.M.I. Liley[6] believes that infants, in utero, trigger some of the physical changes in the mother's body that nourish them. The placenta, considered an organ of the infant, produces many hormones necessary to maintain pregnancy. By producing these substances, unborn infants actively participate and exert some control over their survival. It is claimed that a disproportionate number of disabled children are born to rejecting mothers. It appears that the fetus senses a hostile environment and withdraws, thus causing itself harm.[7] Here we can see an example of the unique spirit of the fetus interpreting and making meaning of his surrounding. Such a response cannot be explained as reflex only.

Science teaches us that the behavior of the fetus is: "an expression of inherited structure (genes, hormones, and environment) and that the diet or illness of the mother can alter that structure, thereby affecting the neuromuscular mechanisms, thus altering behavior."[8]

This hypothesis acknowledges the importance of reflex action in the fetus' behavior but it does not explain the ability of the unborn child to give meaning to a series of events and to initiate a particular response. The ability to respond with meaning transcends the physical and neurological explanation of behavior, although they are its means of expression.

Let us use Kristina—the baby who rejected her mother—as an example. Kristina was, as reported by medical authorities and judged by her parents, a well-developed, normal, healthy infant girl. However, normal, healthy babies suck eagerly for refreshment—either their mother's milk or bottled formula. Kristina chose bottled formula and a stranger's breast milk over her own mother's milk.

What prompted her to do that? Kristina, despite her limited infant capacity, responded with behavior that indicated her state of mind and emotions. She was acting with integrity. Her individual spirit, part of her wholeness, had been wounded, and she would have no more of it! Another baby might have acquiesced; but Kristina was already making a choice, intrinsically preserving her sense of self-worth.

The important point here is that the capacity to respond in this way developed in the womb, before Kristina's birth. The potential for such spirit, or such a capacity to respond as an individual, has to be present at conception in the original cell formation derived from the egg and sperm, as it is an intrinsic dimension of the whole person and thus cannot be added at a later time.

This capacity or spirit gradually matures to keep pace with the physical body and nerves or "inherited structure" of the fetus. It is the third element comprising the triad of body, mind and spirit that begins our existence. All three require nourishment from the beginning of conception to the end of our lives. It might be said that a peaceful, active spirit is the harmony that is partly derived from the integration of the physical and psychological areas of being.

We are again reminded that acceptance by the mother of her pregnancy, and her love and concern, have a bearing on the health and personality of the child. If the child is not accepted, the child will sense this and will enter life at birth with a wounded spirit and a lessened sense of self-worth. Unfortunately, this wound often goes undetected, and so the child is left to grapple with the consequences of this rejection alone.

If all this seems too complex for a developing fetus, consider the fact that laboratory studies have placed the start of awareness in the fetus between the twenty-eighth and thirty-second week. By this time, studies show that the brain's neural circuits are as advanced as those of a newborn infant.

Further, Dr. Verny, quoted in the previous chapter, has acknowledged a third source of communication between mother and child. Compared to the communication channels provided by biology (physiological) and the behavior of the mother, Dr. Verny finds this third channel—which he terms "sympathetic communication"—difficult to define.[9] He uses this term to account for the deeper knowledge the infant acquires while in the womb, such as that which Kristina displayed which cannot be explained physically or biologically.

Elizabeth Noble, in her 1993 book *Primal Connection,* goes further. She claims divine consciousness or illumination exists in the physiological as well as the psychological. Noble cites medical researchers who have raised the question of a "non-physical memory." The brain may work as a tuning device and storage may be outside both the brain and the body.[10]

Dr. Thomas Franz, professor of Counseling Psychology at State University of New York at Buffalo uses the same metaphor of a tuning device to describe his theory of non-verbal vibratory communication experienced by every individual. Franz calls the process entrainment. (Entrainment is a dynamic of nature as pervasive as gravity and involves the process by which one system falls in sync with another.) Dr. Franz claims that the energy of which we are composed acts the same as a tuning fork that vibrates. Such energy vibrations begin to move "in tune" and at the same rate as the person with whom one is in contact. The energy of one complex vibratory individual moves out, affecting the other person, sending messages of which we may be totally unaware.[11] (Examples of this occur when female roommates at college find their menstrual cycles begin to occur at the same time.) Noble expresses this unconscious movement in the following way: "There is a momentum toward wholeness in us all toward the expression of our spirits longing to harmoniously interact with whom we have some connections."[12]

Such terms as sympathetic communication, vibratory exchange of energy, and spiritual interaction, all describe the relationship of the spirit of the mother with the spirit of the fetus in her womb. The spiritual capacity of the infant is further developed as the bond between mother and baby deepens and the child grows. The baby comes to realize that the mother is the source of its sustenance. The mother, in turn, begins to have a sense of the infants unfolding, unique personality. All of this communication is on a deep, non-verbal level. Young children are exceedingly sensitive to emotional and spiritual vibration. It is their chief means of cognition.

Many researchers have studied and documented the profound apathy of hospitalized children who have been left unattended by their mothers, either intentionally or by virtue of circumstances. This is formally recognized as the failure-to-thrive syndrome. This often seen condition also underscores the need of the spirit (ability to respond as an individual) for emotional support. Lack of such support weakens the spirit and the body. Infants who are so deprived have no energy left with which to develop their own resources for individual response, as it is too soon for such development to take place without the support of the familiar presence of the mother. Thus, the infant remains listless and apathetic. We must, then, draw the conclusion that the loving presence of the mother nourishes all three areas of the infant's development in the womb and at birth, and therefore, influences the infant's personality development.

Spirit And Sexuality

The spirit is an important factor in the development of our sexuality as it is an intrinsic part of our existence from conception. If an individual spirit is not present at conception, the cells will produce a biological automaton rather than a human being. Peerbolte claims the spiritual self to be invisible in the field of attraction between the sperm and egg.[13]

Our spirit is the inner core of our being from which the integrity of the person is developed. It contributes to our ability to make independent responses as male and female to our life experiences. It requires support, both by example and by the provision of information, especially during the early development of the person. It gives meaning to our individual uniqueness. It allows us to transcend our ego in order to attain the self-knowledge that is the basis of self-love. In fact, without spirit there can be no self-love as the individual has failed to find the Source of Love dwelling within the individual self. In such knowledge lies maturity, especially with regard to our sense of masculinity and femininity. Such a mature sense of gender influences our sexual behavior. So often, a lack of self-love and self-esteem is the basis for promiscuous sexual behavior, especially during adolescence. This type of behavior is often chosen by a child (or an adult) who lacking unconditional love, seeks affection but lacks the self-respect (self-love) to use good judgment. Such lack of self-respect can lead to an inability to form an intimate relationship in adulthood. "During our development, the sensual and spiritual elements of the human personality fuse, and as one mode receives, the other will also be affected; when one mode is deprived, the other is also deprived."[14]

The spirit as an integral part of the individual is both conscious and unconscious. It forms the basis of what is often called intuition. It interacts with our thinking (conceptual) and feeling (sensate) abilities to influence our behavior. The uniqueness of the individual is fostered because the same psychological factors impinge on each personality differently depending on the meaning given to these factors by the individual spirit.

Our behavior and our sexuality—the sense of being masculine or feminine—are affected by the deprivation of the spirit. We cannot become whole beings when deprivation of the spirit occurs. Our sexuality can then only then become, partly or wholly, an expression of physical need. A mature spirit gives to our sexuality a fuller meaning, directing it toward another in its natural human expression. Thomas Keating, a Benedictine monk, describes our sexuality as "embodied energy that desires to be in relationship with all of life on a physical, psychological and emotional plane."[15] Our sexuality can only be nurtured to maturity by unconditional love—both human and Divine, especially in early life.

Spirit And Children

This holistic view of our sexuality, if presented to children in their early years, would help to make them aware of their ability to cope with and overcome life's challenges. It would form a basis for a mature understanding of the erotic aspect of their sexuality.

Development of the spirit in the context of the whole person encourages us to be independent, creative and real. It is a basis upon which children form their own values. A warm, loving relationship encourages the spirit to grow and allows children to be free to be themselves. If the spirit of a child is badly wounded or untended during pregnancy or in the early years, then as an adult, this person will see through a glass darkly and will be unable to grasp the light of his/her individual truth.

The existence of the spirit is too often lost in the plethora of information that passes for education. Sometimes it is ignored, sometimes denied. Often the spirit is misformed or disabled by the overzealousness of organized religion. Religious beliefs must be built on, and must be accompanied by respect for, the natural spirit of the individual.

Dr. Robert Coles, a psychiatrist and professor at Harvard, has made a comprehensive study of the spiritual life of children.[16] In his interviews with the children, Coles found that they held their own diverse and individual sense of the spiritual which did not necessarily coincide with the beliefs or practice of their parents. What was established by this study is that children have an evolving spiritual side to their nature—an inner life that must be respected. Coles' research verified children's instinctive knowledge of God in many forms. Children are linked with the Divine. As they develop, even as babies, that link or that "thread" can become weakened unless it is nurtured by unconditional love. Often, by the time these persons reach adulthood, the connection has been almost obliterated. Not only have these adults not received unconditional love in the period of their infant individuation, but the resultant lack of self-love has prevented them from nurturing that part of themselves that is of the spirit.

The existence of a spiritual life in children is illustrated by the story of Joey, a three-year old who was seemingly preoccupied with death.

Joey's mother, early in her pregnancy, had experienced uterine bleeding to such an extent that a miscarriage seemed inevitable. However, after a time, normal development of the fetus began to proceed and Joey was delivered at term.

One of the possible reasons offered by her obstetrician for the excessive bleeding was that Joey's mother had conceived twins and one of the fetuses had miscarried. During her pregnancy, Joey's mother had been grieving without quite knowing why. The obstetrician's explanation gave her some peace and a reasonable interpretation for her sense of loss. Joey's mother, a warm, loving person, had been very respectful of Joey's unique pattern of growth toward autonomy and identity. She had worked part-time since Joey was about two years of age, but continued to breastfeed him until age three.

Joey had been busy with his development as a near-four-year-old, which included adjusting to separation from his mother via school and new playmates. Instinctively, Joey seems to know that he must give up something of his old life to begin something new. This could be one of the reasons for his present preoccupation with death. He has asked such questions as "How old do you have to be to die?" He has also related the following dream to his mother: "I was searching and looking for someone who was important to me. I was looking and I was very sad. When I found him, he was dead. I was feeling very sad. Then I woke up." This story was not prompted by any previous conversation or discussion. Rather it is Joey's way of making meaning of his own life experiences.

While playing in the bathtub, Joey again brought up the subject of death, saying to his mother, "Mom, we're dead." His mother replied, playing along, "Well we must be happy because we are together in heaven." Joey thought for a moment and then said, "Mom, I am going to be very good and when I die, I will go straight to heaven, and you know Mom, when you are in heaven, you never die." "Who told you that?" his mother queried. Joey asserted confidently, "I just know it."

His mother made no reply to these assertions so surprised was she at the notion of goodness, reward, and eternity implied in her young son's statement—beliefs that she had never attempted to teach him.

The experiences of Joey and Kristina lend credence to the existence of an inner sense (or spirit) in children that reacts to their womb experiences.

Many books have been written about the physical and psychological care of children but few, if any, have addressed the nurturing of their innate spiritual capacity. Although the unconditional love of parents provides most of the necessary nurturing for the spirit, it is important for parents to explore the meaning their children are making of their own experiences. The revelations Joey made to his mother would not have been made had she not continually respected Joey's perceptions and growing belief system. Such revelations certainly add to the sense of intimacy in the parental relationship, teaching both child and parent the joys of love.

Thomas Hora, a metapsychiatrist, refers to such joy in his definition of spiritual identity. He asks:

What is a strong spiritual identity? It is in proportion to our love of purity, order, harmony, peace, assurance and gratitude. The more we appreciate these qualities of consciousness, the stronger we become spiritually…. The normal condition of man is to be joyful…behavior has to manifest joy and freedom.[17]

In brief...

❖ The third essential part of our whole being is spirit.

❖ The spiritual component of our being is present at conception. It, together with the physical and psychological components of our being, is nurtured by unconditional love.

❖ Our spirit is that part of us that develops and makes fast the thread by which each of us is connected to the divine.

❖ The spirit is manifested by one's individual's uniqueness and singular ability to develop a special view of his or her experience. Our spirit can transcend the physical-neurological expression of behavior.

❖ The growth of the spirit is essential to our development into a mature, sexual adult as it is a crucial component in the development of self-love. Without a love of self, which requires the integration of body, mind, and spirit, mature sexuality is not possible.

Chapter 7—Endnotes

1 Claremont de Castellijo, Irene, M.D., *Knowing Women*, Harper Colophon Books, Harper & Row, New York, NY, 1974

2 Ibid

3 Needleman, Jacob, "Questions of the Heart", *Noetic Science Review*, No. 26, Summer, 1993, p.5. Sausalito, CA

4 Noble, Elizabeth, *Primal Connection*, Simon & Schuster, New York, N. Y., 1993

5 Jourard, Sidney, M., *The Transparent Self*, Von Nostrand Reinhold Co., Inc., Florida, 1971, revised edition

6 Liley, M.M.I., M.D., as cited by Schwartz, *The World of the Unborn*, Marek Publishers, New York, NY 1980

7 Stott, Dennis, follow-up study from "Birth of Effects of Prenatal Stress, Developmental Medicine", *Child Neurology*, vol. 15, pp. 770-787, London, England, 1973

8 Lewontin, Richard, *Human Diversity*, Scientific American Library, Scientific American Books, W. H. Freeman & Co., New York, N. Y., 1982

9 Verny, Thomas, M. D., with John Kelly, *The Secret Life of the Unborn*, Summit Books, Division of Simon & Schuster, New York, N. Y., 1981

10 Noble, Elizabeth, op. cit, pp. 65-67

11 Franz, Thomas, M. D., professor of Counseling Psychology at State University of New York at Buffalo, (personal interview) 9/21/92

12 Noble, op cit, p.67

13 Peerbolte, Lietaert, M., *Prenatal Dynamics*, Leyden, Netherlands, 1954

14 Arraj, James, *St. John of the Cross and Dr. C. G. Jung*, Inner Growth Books, Chiloquin, Ohio, 1986

15 Keating, Thomas, "Contemplative Spirituality and Sexuality", *Contemplative Outreach News*, Vol. 7, Fall, 1993

16 Coles, Robert, M. D., *Spiritual Life of Children*, Houghton, Mifflin, New York, N.Y., 1990

17 Hora, Thomas, *Dialogues in Metapsychiatry*, Seabury Press, New York, N.Y., 1975

Holistic Birth—A 3-Year Developmental Process

The biological birth of the human infant and the psychological birth of the individual are not coincident in time. The former is a dramatic, observable and well-circumscribed event; the latter, a slowly unfolding intrapsychic process.[1]

Margaret S. Mahler, M.D.
Director of Research,
Masters' Children's Hospital,
New York City

Our child's brain may have its limits set genetically, but it rests within our ability to stimulate this brain before and after birth in order to allow the brain to grow to its fullest potential.[2]

Mortimer Rosen, M.D.
Lynn Rosen, EdD

The reader, at this point, has gained some idea of the intimate interaction of our physical, psychological, and spiritual modes of being—from the moment of conception throughout pregnancy—and how this intrapsychic process influences the formation of our sexual identity, even at the earliest stages of development. Nature has timed the sequence of developmental events carefully. It is our responsibility to be attuned to and knowledgeable about these events so that we may cooperate with and support—rather than thwart—their natural occurrences. The next step of our journey is to examine how this developmental triad affects the infant's birth and early life. However, the reader should bear in mind the intended scope of this book, which makes it possible to emphasize only those physical, psychological, and spiritual influences that clarify the connection between that triad and our identity as masculine or feminine. Of particular importance are the concepts that our sexuality encompasses all three components, and that parents do affect its development.

Thus, this book is not meant to be a comprehensive guide to the growth and development of the newborn infant or the care of the pregnant mother. Rather, this book sets forth the sequence of and influences on the development of our gender/sexual identity from conception to age three.

As Mahler points out in the beginning quote, the psychological birth of the child is a slowly unfolding process. At birth, the infant is not a blank slate on which parents impose a script but neither is its primal identity fully formed.[3] To promote optimal development in all three spheres of being, in the early three years, it is essential that a mother forge a continuous, positive, accepting relationship with her child from conception, throughout pregnancy, and the birth process, until approximately thirty-six months of age. Such a relationship and positive environment will encourage an individuated sexual identity in the child, who will then have a firm foundation upon which to begin to build a separate existence from the mother, gradually maturing toward wholeness.

Great Expectations

Rather than the beginning of life, birth can be viewed as a transitional time when environmental needs of the infant change and a time when an accepting, loving relationship is vital. We have been educated to view birth as ended when the infant emerges from the womb. Not so. The birth of the whole individual usually will take up to approximately three years. At birth, the unique individual who has been carried for nine months in the womb of the mother enters the outside world of the parents with certain rights and expectations, among which is the expectation that the intimate relationship that has been formed during pregnancy will continue. When it doesn't, some of the infant's inherent potential is lost.

We are social beings. Each child is born with social impulses. Emotional hunger, says Dr. Ribble is an "urge as defined and compelling as the need for food."[4] The capacity for psychologically healthy relationships in adulthood begins with the first relationship of mother and child. Other influences enter into our growth to emotional maturity, but the presence of an accepting mother is basic and primary to such development in every sense of the word.

The time of birth to approximately three years (depending on the individual and the circumstances) is a time when the child's sense of self as good and important (a sense begun in the womb) is strengthened and made firm. Such a foundation is necessary for the development of a healthy sense of sexual identity, whether male or female. An intimate relationship with the one who has been central to the first nine months of life activates the feelings of the baby. Touching, soothing and holding stimulate the baby's physical and psychological processes. Such a relationship of love and nurture continues the development of the nervous system to full functioning, thus fostering within each child an individual personality. (Table 8-1 presents a summary of the influence of care giving on the early development of the nervous system.)

Modern women have become confused about the importance of their relationship with their infants, and the information that is generally provided to them contradicts their most basic instincts. Society—especially those in the realms of the medical community and the workplace—tells mothers that others can safely assume care of their infant, especially once the child reaches four months of age, with little risk of negative consequences.

Instinctively, though, mothers feel the need of their children for their presence; that is why those who must make a decision about returning to work often feel so conflicted. Then, too, many mothers lack adequate knowledge of their infant's many needs, which, in turn, makes it easier for them to dismiss their instincts as backward notions in a progressive, daycare-oriented society.

There is a widespread belief that if infants are properly fed and protected from cold and infection, they will develop as fully in body and mind as their native endowment or heritage warrants. That is the emphasis of most medical care. Consider too, the elements of childcare emphasized in advertisements: cleanliness, diapering, weight gain, and formula feeding. These are important, but the concept of whole health is not addressed at all.

Relevant research on the holistic needs of infants is not appropriately emphasized in the education of new parents, so little is known of the importance of psychological development in postnatal care. Decisions regarding the care of the infant are often made almost exclusively on the basis of economic factors and reflect the mother's lack of trust in her own judgment vis-à-vis societal pressures. In order to fulfill the needs of infants at critical times, women need research-based information to believe what their innate sense tells them is correct—that their children need them in order to grow to be loving adults. Armed with that knowledge, parents can sort out the myths perpetuated by the media and consumer advertising and be free to act on their instincts.

In light of this, let us consider the whole child and how this wholeness is nurtured by a mother's continuous care, at least until the child reaches the age of three years. For the purpose of clarity, each area of growth—physical, psychological and spiritual—will be considered in separate chapters, although in reality all three are intricately interwoven.

Sexuality And Maturation Of The Nervous System

Modern research supports the close interrelationship of our sexuality and the development of the brain and central nervous system. As stated in Chapter 5, the nervous system does not complete its initial development until approximately eighteen months after birth. Providing a nurturing love during this critical period of neurological development fosters healthy functioning. It is the first of several critical periods for the establishment of sexual identity.

Recall that the brain and other parts of the nervous system grow faster before birth and in the early years of life than muscles, genitals, or other body components. That is why a two-month old fetus has a head almost half its body length. Three weeks after conception, the brain stem begins to form.

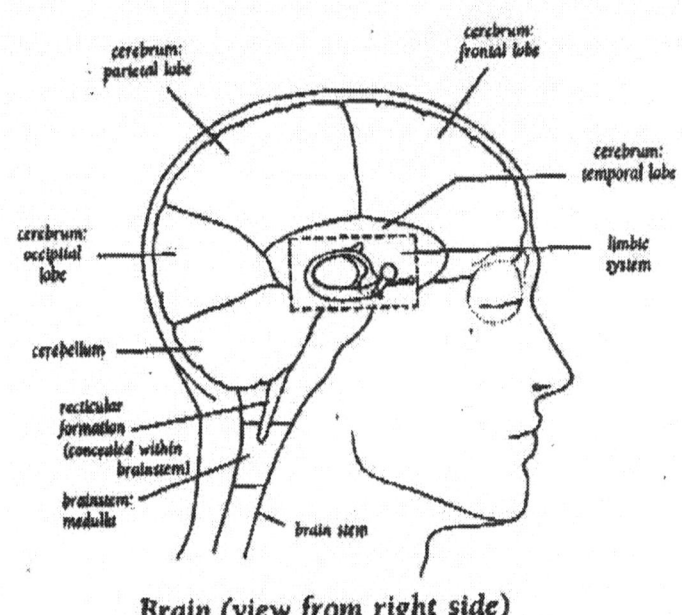

Brain (view from right side)

Figure 8-1 Located at the top of our spine (just below our ears), the brain stem is the oldest part of our brain. In evolutionary terms, it is virtually identical to the brain of a reptile; hence, scientists refer to it as the "reptilian" brain. It houses reticular formation, which alerts the brain to incoming data from the body and governs basic activities like consciousness, breathing, and heart rate. (Maguire, Care and Feeding of the Brain, p. 5)

At birth, the brain has developed to one-quarter of its adult weight. Within six months after birth, a child's brain weight is doubled. Maguire describes the importance of the brain:

> In contrast to the wonder it arouses, the physical brain itself looks comically insignificant. About three pounds in weight and the size of two fists, it resembles an upscaled jellied walnut. But that jellied walnut has been 500 million years in the making, and it is by far the most remarkable organ in our body, both architecturally and functionally. More than anything else, giving it the attention it deserves requires appreciating why it is so extraordinary.[5]

Although the newborn baby has almost all the neurons (nerve cells) its brain will ever hold, they have yet to form a subtle mesh of links—the mesh that helps transform this kit of parts into a fully integrated mechanism. Scientists used to think neurons linked up haphazardly. Now they believe the nervous system includes chemically coded specifications determining where neurons latch on to one another. The forging of these links hold a key to the maturing of the brain (see Figure 8-2). It is as though the infant needs to experience nurturing care so as to strengthen appropriate connections in the maze of brain circuitry.

In a recent Canadian study, researchers found that early nurturing contributed to an increase in synapses (neural connectors). They also found more receptors for growth hormones and the neurotransmitter NMDA that is crucial to learning. "There is evidence for a direct relationship between maternal care and hippocampal development and spatial learning in adulthood."[6]

How The Brain Matures

Different areas of the brain grow at varying times and at varying rates, before and after birth. The following diagram shows which parts of the cerebral cortex are earliest and latest to mature. Areas that a baby needs first, such as centers controlling sensation and movement, are first to mature, but there is great variation within these areas—for example, sensitivity to bright light precedes detailed vision by many months.[7]

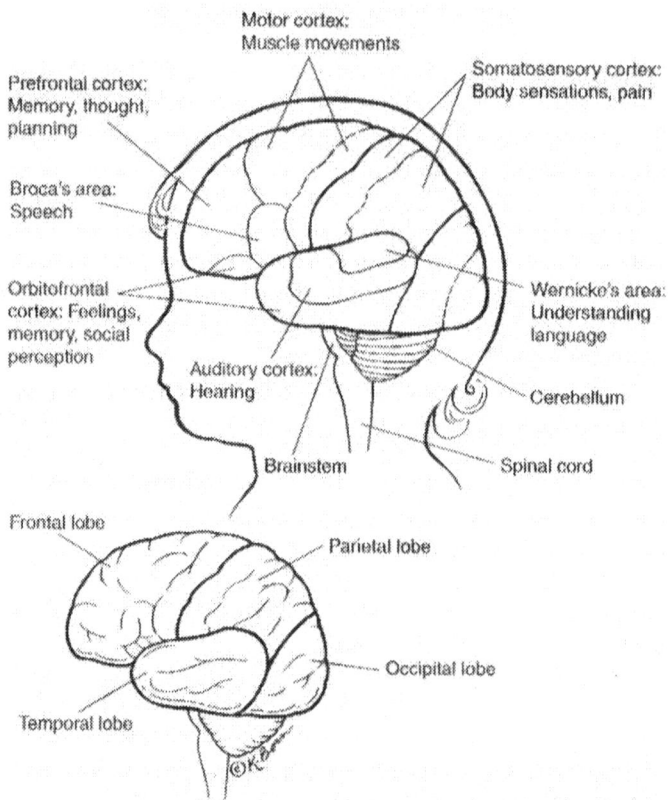

Figure 8-2 The Cerebral Cortex—The cortex is divided into specialized areas, although these regions do not have any fixed borders or "walls" around them. (A Good Start in Life—Norbert Herschkowitz, M.D. and Elinore Chapman Herschkowitz, p. 113)

According to Maguire,[8] male and female brains are structured differently. Both sexes have a right and a left hemisphere, sections of the brain that govern different activities. To explain briefly, the cortex of the cerebrum's left hemisphere is thought to govern analytical functions, such as language comprehension, speaking, computing, and judging time and sequence. By contrast, the cortex of the cerebrum's right hemisphere is mostly responsible for such imaginative activities as recognizing faces, reconstructing melodies, and visualizing images. However, Maguire reminds us that such strict division of activity is not scientifically correct, and that most of the mental processes require both hemispheres working together.

In females, the cortex of the left hemisphere tends to be thicker. As a consequence, women are generally better at language skills and penmanship than men are, and excel at other fine motor skills as well. In males, the cortex of the right hemisphere is thicker, so men are generally better at spatial tasks and large muscle skills.

Neurosurgeon George Ojeman of the University of Washington has produced scores of detailed maps of people's individual language centers. Not only has he found sexual differences but has also determined that instead of the same sites laid down more or less in everyone, they are laid down is subtly different places in the brain. Another score for the uniqueness of the individual.

This does not mean that either sex cannot learn the skills of the other. Rather, it means that men and women are cast in complementary roles and they can learn from and help each other.

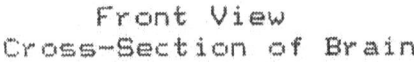

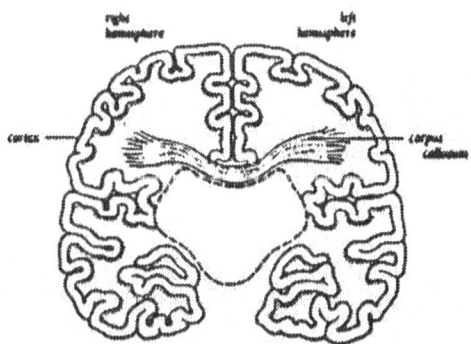

Figure 8-3 Maguire—Care and Feeding o f the Brain

Another difference scientists have found is that the network of fibers that connect the two hemispheres (known as the corpus collosum) is larger in the female brain than in the male brain. This structural difference has two effects:

1. Women generally recover more quickly from brain damage than men do; and
2. As the brain develops, it becomes more specialized.

Women reach puberty earlier, so it is assumed that they have less time for specialization. Because it takes longer for men to reach puberty, their brain becomes more specialized. The stronger corpus collosum in the female brain may explain woman's intuition, as she may be able to communicate more quickly between hemispheres. The compartmentalized male brain is thought to be better suited for focusing with precision on a "limited number of relevant details." Thus, male individuals, as they have more specialized brain hemispheres, are more frequently victims of dyslexia, stuttering, autism and hyperactivity.[9]

The hormones that are responsible for the development of sexual characteristics in the womb—estrogen and testosterone—also influence brain tissues and the brain's transmission system (reception of stimuli, motor reflexes, etc.), thus facilitating the brain's operation. But again, there are differences.

Many researchers believe that sex hormones produced early in fetal development...as well as after birth, "literally sex the brain"...says Bruce McEwen of the New York Rockefeller University, a neuroendocrinologist.

> Males produce testosterone from the 3rd to the 6th month of gestation. Another burst is released just after birth and then one final spurt at the onset of puberty—roughly coinciding with the time boys begin to surpass girls in math. What is more, males with an abnormality that makes their cells insensitive to testosterone's effects have cognitive profiles identical to girls. Their verbal IQ is higher than in normal males and their performance IQ (correlated with mechanical ability) is inferior to that of normal males.[10]

It is interesting to note that recent studies by LeVay of the Salk Institute have indicated that specific clusters of brain cells are invariably larger in heterosexual men than in homosexual men. However, no corroborating research has been completed as yet to verify this finding. Nonetheless, it is interesting to speculate whether this difference might be apparent in the womb, or at least during the first three years of life when brain development is proceeding so rapidly, and what factors might contribute to it.

Dr. Silber, author of *The Male* feels the brain is the most important sex organ as it is the hypothalamus that controls the interplay of hormonal events in the female's menstrual cycle and, in the male, the steady release of neurotransmitters that stimulate the testicles to make hormones and sperm. (It should be remembered that sex hormone levels do not "predict" a person's sexual behavior or interest. Such behaviors or interest are psychologically based.)

Learning about the typical patterns of sexual development during childhood, can help parents (or prospective parents) become more effective in helping their children develop and learn about sexuality. There is a great deal of scientific evidence that refutes the position that men and women are interchangeable in all respects. They are equal—not interchangeable—and that is an important fact for children to learn.

Breastfeeding, Development Of The Nervous System, Bonding, And Beyond

If, as science tells us, the nervous system of the child (including the brain), with its subsequent influence on sexual development, does not mature fully until about eighteen months of age, we can easily see how important it is to care for the infant properly during this period so that maximal development is achieved and an intact sexual identity is formed. As Ribble notes,

> The infant may have an excellent endowment in the actual protoplasm of his brain, yet may never acquire full use of it without stimulus and direction…first feeling experiences stimulate an innate capacity of the brain of the baby to associate inner needs with outer satisfaction. This gives an important impetus to the evolution of the mental life.[11]

Initially, the infant's physical needs include stimulation, sucking, food, oxygen, cleanliness, and rest in comfortable surroundings. But, delivery to the senses of the infant must have proper intensity and occur at the right time, otherwise, his or her inherent openness to experience will change abruptly into an attitude of diffused defense.

At birth, the greatest environmental change that occurs is the absence of familiar stimuli. Newborn infants must instead adapt to a host of unfamiliar, sometimes noxious stimuli, all characterizing the world outside the womb. For the infant, there was a certain constancy in the womb which is no longer present at birth However, the warmth of the mother's arms and the sound of her voice, though somewhat changed, are familiar and reassuring to the infant. If the father has also been communicating with the infant in the womb, then his voice will be a welcome sound also.

Drs. Marshal Klaus and John Kennell (at Case Western Reserve Medical School in 1976) are well known for their observance and reporting of a specific bonding ritual between human mother and her newborn infant. This is often frustrated and short-circuited by technological birth and routine separation of the infant from mother after birth. Direct eye-to-eye contact, extensive holding and touching, maternal soothing and crooning sounds, and mutual smiling appear to be crucial in orienting infants to their new surroundings. Mothers who were allowed sixteen hours of extra contact with their babies after birth were reluctant to leave their infants up to one year of age. Such contact helps to establish intimacy, a basis for adult sexual intimacy. The so-called dance of the mother and baby is a forerunner of the dance of sexual union.

A five-year follow up of Klaus and Kennell's study (which is still ongoing) has shown that those infants who have a greater degree of intimate contact with mothers during the hours and days immediately postpartum, achieve developmental milestones significantly earlier. At age five, the IQ, as well as the speech and language comprehension of these children was significantly superior to those of the control group who had a lesser degree of intimate contact with their mothers.[12]

LeBoyer also reports that intimate contact with the mother results in children who are adroit with both hands, who begin to talk at an early age, and who experience less difficulty with toilet training and self-feeding than do those deprived of such contact.

Being in the arms of the mother, at birth and thereafter, more closely simulates the warmth of the womb than any other extrauterine experience. Being able to suck while being held close to warm, human skin (thereby satisfying both hunger and stimulation needs) the child is allowed to develop within the context of a pleasant sexual ambiance. At the same time, the infant is developing trust in another human. There are no barriers at this time to that trusting relationship.

Nature supplies mothers with the necessary "tools" to meet their infant's first needs. About three weeks before birth the mother experiences a sharp decline in her progesterone levels and a sharp increase in estrogen. This dramatic rise in estrogen levels triggers maternal behavior. The estrogen level is not sustained, however, without the close contact with the infant that is necessary for bonding. This natural process is largely unknown to parents, as is the fact that bonding is the prelinguistic method of communication for mother and child in which language skills have their root.

Through breastfeeding, nature offers an excellent means of fulfilling the infant's needs on several levels during this critical growth period including the physical needs of stimulation, sucking, food, and comfort. Indeed, if the infant's first feeding experiences are pleasurable, this will contribute to a sense of satisfaction that has far-reaching effects.

The mouth is fundamentally an organ of touch. Its nerve supply comes directly from the brain through five different cranial nerves. The intense neurological stimulation of suckling (the lips are well-endowed with sensory nerve endings) combines with the satisfaction of milk to send messages to the brain that are interpreted as pleasurable and that activate sexual reflexes.[13]

Through breastfeeding, nature has provided the infant with easy-to-digest food at just the right temperature, combined with sucking stimulation and comfort. Modern technology, bottle and formula manufacturers, and frequently, the mother's need to return to work have too often eroded the mother's confidence in this natural process, thus denying the infant the inherent benefits of breastfeeding.

Some mothers reject breastfeeding because they fear their sexual response to such an intimate act. A few women even experience orgasm while breastfeeding. Such feelings are natural and can be pleasurable depending on the knowledge and training of the mother.

Many mothers reject breastfeeding because at the outset they feel clumsy and inexperienced. It is well to remember that mothers and babies have communicated for several months before birth, and they will eventually surmount any difficulties, achieving a level of comfort with the process that satisfies them both. (The LaLeche League, which serves mothers all over the world, was formed just for the purpose of helping mothers at this time).

There are other advantages of breastfeeding. Breast milk is better suited for the infant's digestive system than formula or cows' milk, with less protein and more lactose. Indeed, cows' milk was never designed for human babies, but for calves with four stomachs!

The high protein content is the main reason for diluting cows' milk and then the other nutrients decrease proportionately. Adding sugar is damaging to the intestines. Some of the proteins in cows' milk differ from those in breast milk. Cows' milk does not supply secretory IGA which is of vital importance in the first 14 days of life and its influence lasts through adulthood.

The relatively high level of linolenic acid in breast milk leads to better DNA production, higher brain (cortex) DNA levels and better developmental status at 18 months. These fatty acids are essential for normal cell membranes, for normal brain and neurological development, and for many other reactions involved in the fine tuning of the way the body functions and develops. Human milk also contains more cholesterol than cows' milk. Cholesterol is thought to be important for development of brain and neurons.[14]

The content and amount of breast milk changes naturally and automatically in response to the needs of the baby, and is easily available. Breast milk contains the antibodies of the mother and thus helps to ward off infection and prevent most allergies in the first six months. In fact, nature is so finely attuned to the infant's needs that a good supply of protein content is provided as the baby initiates feeding, and, as the baby continues to suck, lactose content increases, providing a suitable dessert!

To return specifically to the development of the brain and nervous system, Dr. James Prescott, in his work at John Hopkins University Hospital, states,

The role of olfaction [sense of smelling] is of particular significance in affectional bonding where extended breastfeeding (2-3 years) results in the encoding of woman's natural body odors in the developing brain which becomes intimately associated with pleasure bonding with the mother (woman). The failure to develop olfactory pleasure encoding in the brain results in…aversion to women's natural body odors [and] in touch aversion behaviors.[15]

It would seem safe to say that breastfeeding helps the infant to feel at home with the feel and smell of his own body as well as that of another, encoding the brain for future intimate relationships.

Breastfeeding also helps to develop the myelin sheathing of the nerves (see Table 8-1). Such sheathing acts as an insulation. It protects the nerves and improves synaptic transmission from twelve to twenty times faster; another factor in the evolution of mental capacity. Because eye development is incomplete at birth, early eye stimulation is essential to retaining vision.[16] (See Figure 8-2) For example, the retina in the eye is not properly developed at birth, and the nerves coursing from the eyes through the brain lack insulating sheaths of myelin at birth. About two weeks after birth, the baby will look at a face. They are learning to perceive. By six weeks, both eyes can focus on one object. By three months, the infant has a full adult field of vision. Not only does breastfeeding help form the myelin sheathing for neurons, the actual act of breastfeeding provides visual stimulation, completing the process!

British scientists, after reviewing vast amounts of research on breastfeeding and disease, suggest that the benefits of mother's milk extend well beyond infancy. Breastfed babies, compared to those who are bottlefed, experience fewer bouts with pneumonia, middle ear infections, respiratory infections, and spinal meningitis. Bottle feeding is associated with as much as a 16 percent higher incidence of such illnesses as flu and spinal meningitis. In fact, bottle feeding is known to be associated with immune system disorders, diabetes, chronic liver disease, ulcerative colitis, celiac disease and Crohn's disease, many of which develop later in life. Modern medicine and formula manufacturers, in encouraging mothers to bottle feed their infants, are breaking the bond between mother and child and depriving the child of a natural health-giving source. Very often breastfeeding is not emphasized in childbirth classes in an effort to leave the choice to the mother. All facts should be presented so the mother can make an informed choice.

We see very clearly how breastfeeding easily meets the physical needs of the infant. It provides nutritious food, on demand, that nourishes the body, thereby stimulating the brain and nervous system development that is important for the infant's developing sexual identity. It protects the infant from disease when most vulnerable; it provides the sucking stimulation necessary for speech development, and it continues the same intuitive, preverbal communication between mother and baby that began in the womb. It is estimated that only about 5 percent of women cannot breastfeed. It is often attitude and determination that affects successful breastfeeding.

The reader should not, however, assume that breastfeeding is the total answer to mother's responsibility. Margaret Mead's studies help to underscore this point. Her studies of the natives of Bali and Samoa have revealed that, although infants are allowed to breastfeed on demand and thus have their instinctual hunger and sucking needs consistently satisfied, emotional ties are not nurtured in these societies.

Infants might be cared for by any member of the family, even breastfed by another mother, and emotional ties to one person are not developed. Too close ties to the mother are often ridiculed. Since social relationships are based mainly on food satisfaction and protection against strangers outside the group, they are unable, as they develop, to form good parental relationships. Instead, sex drive is in evidence at an early age and supplants an ability to maintain a relationship otherwise. When taken out of their family group, these children failed to function and became depressed.[17]

This research supports the need for a consistent, good relationship with the mother until the child's own identity is established and s/he can begin to relate to others.

To me, there is a parallel to be drawn between the Bali and Samoa approach to child care and the common practice of subjecting children to a number of caretakers at an early age, often without the benefit of breastfeeding. Could the alarming trends developing in the United States—such as failure to learn, early inappropriate sexual activity, and teenage suicide (up 300 percent between 1955 and 1975)—be the result of our practice of separating mother and child at too early an age? Other researchers agree with me that the connection is all too evident.

Dr. Mary Giffen, Medical Director of the North Shore Mental Health Association in Illinois, describes a "typical" suicidal adolescent as

> one who is likely to be a teenager who very early in life was literally separated from important relationships or who never experienced a real trusting relationship. Thus he remained alone to cope with the stress and strain of growing up.... It is essential that we begin a loving relationship with our children from the earliest possible moment. We must realize that the suicidal impulse can be ingrained within the first few months of life.[18]

Sexual Development vs. Violence

When we analyze how our children are developing, we are apt to say, "he is good at math, like his father" or "she gets her good disposition from her mother." What we now know is that the traits we are distinguishing in our children are not only a matter of heredity but are a result of our behavior as parents, especially the environment created by the mother. The mother's environment, of course, especially the degree to which she is nurtured, affects her ability to provide the crucial positive environment for her child.

In the preceding section, we mentioned the influence of bonding—or its lack—on the rate of suicide. Suicide is a violence to self. Violence to others is also endemic in our society. Dr. Prescott, quoted earlier, connects violence and parent-infant relationships as follows:

> ...the deprivation of physical affection in human relationships, beginning in the parent-infant relationship...constitutes the greatest source of physical violence in societies. The sensory neurobiological mechanism of physical pleasure are mediated (brought about) by the somesthetic (touch) and vestibular (movement) sensory systems where the cerebellum has been proposed as a master integrating and regulating system for sensory-emotional, psychological and spiritual experience.[19]

In other words, pleasant physical stimuli at an early age affects the brain mechanism which controls our emotional and spiritual experiences. Further confirmation is found in another of Dr. Prescott's findings—one I find of extreme importance.

> ...the neural circuits of the brain that mediate pleasure, control and regulate the neural circuits of the brain that mediate violence. When the pleasure circuits of the brain are damaged through incomplete development due to somatosensory affectional deprivation, then uncontrolled violence is the consequence.[20]

In other words, either pleasure or violence can be conveyed by the same neural circuits of the brain. When pleasant feelings are absent, feelings of violence become predominant. Could teenage suicide and violence be reduced in our society by more mothers breastfeeding and parents loving their children?

The Samuels, Mike and Nancy (authors of The Well Baby Book) sum up the infant-parent interaction very well.

At the most basic level, the more mothers and other people look at, touch, hold and talk to babies, the more the babies will explore, vocalize, manipulate and learn. Real direct attention develops in babies the confident expectancy that their actions will affect the environment and produce results. (I am important.) This attitude is important not just to specific behavior, but to all learning. The sense of competence thus instilled goes beyond intellectual learning to social and emotional adaptation patterns. Positive patterning increases babies ability to deal with frustration and stress. Early stimulation may partially arouse the body's stress system (the adrenocortico-costeroid mechanism) and this experience may produce better ability to handle later stress experiences.[21]

Spiritual Development Of The Infant

Trust and autonomy grow out of the nurturance of the infant's spirit. We will deal with trust development in the next chapter. Here we need to return to the very primitive form of the spirit which is formed in the womb—formation evidenced by the response of the infant, Kristina, as related in previous chapters. Her behavior was reflective of responsive learning and a strong spirit of integrity formed even before birth. A spirit of integrity means that the infant has an essential capacity to respond in a way that preserves not only uniqueness but also wholeness. Infants are unique in their capacity to respond and make meaning of their experiences. The mother-infant relationship is central to the development of that capacity. Giffen describes bonding as:

> ...a matter of responsiveness of a magic person who always comes when the baby cries, who cuddles, soothes and reassures him, who always knows what the baby wants and gives it immediately.[22]

The spirit of the infant develops out of this "magic" responsiveness; the baby has the sense that he or she has some control over the environment. As pointed out by Giffen, out of this sense of competence and ability to respond grows the child's ability to love. The infant, loved unconditionally, learns also to love. This is not love in the romantic sense that is so popular in today's world, but an ability, arising out of having been loved, to go out to others. All of this occurs on an almost mystical preverbal level that stays with the person all their adult life. You have undoubtedly met people whom you instinctively liked and trusted, even before you knew much about them. (See vibratory communication—Chapter 7) The spirit of such people has been fostered by love, and they give off a loving aura that makes the other person with whom they are communicating feel good about his or herself.[23] What a wonderful treasure to develop! In addition, our spirit is the connecting thread to the Divine that Castelljo speaks of. It is the part of us that is able to respond to Divine Love. To neglect the development of the spirit in a child creates a hindrance in the development of his unique personality.

In Leight's definition of our sexuality as "the total of who you are, what you believe and how you respond," (see Chapter 9) we see now that the spirit—our ability to respond—enters into our sexuality. We must admit that this wholeness begins with the mother-infant relationship in the womb and continues with a similar relationship until about the age of three years. The physical, psychological, and spiritual areas of development are inextricably interwoven to produce a whole sexual being. Following birth, physical contact with the mother takes the place of the prenatal physical connection of the fetus, when the child was like an organ of the mother's body. Breastfeeding helps the infant feel comfortable in familiar surroundings. Breastfeeding makes it easy for the mother to foster a child's holistic development. The father, too, in his affectionate, protective treatment of the mother and child, contributes to the bonding of all three members of the family (see Chapter 10).

By the age of three years, or thereabouts, normal infants, properly parented, have learned that they have control over their body functions and locomotion, and that they have a separate identity from their mothers. Moreover, they are able to form an image of their mothers in their minds when she is not present which helps to prevent a sense of loss. They feel good about themselves as important, they know what sex they are, and they have pretty much mastered their world of development and are ready to explore a larger world—gradually.

The basic ability to love is fostered in such a developmental scheme. So often we try to teach the ability to love in our school-aged children through a system of discipline and rewards, ignoring the fact that in the womb and during the first three years of life, we have either fostered or thwarted such capability.

Of course, the reader will understand that the positive relationship we have been describing should not end at three years of age. Rather, it should be allowed to continue, but with the gradual introduction of other stimuli, so that what the child has learned from the parents, especially the mother, will be transferred to relationships with others. Activities, such as two half-days a week at nursery school, swimming lessons, music classes, and participation in parties with neighborhood children, all gradually introduce a child to his or her expanding world in doses that can be assimilated.

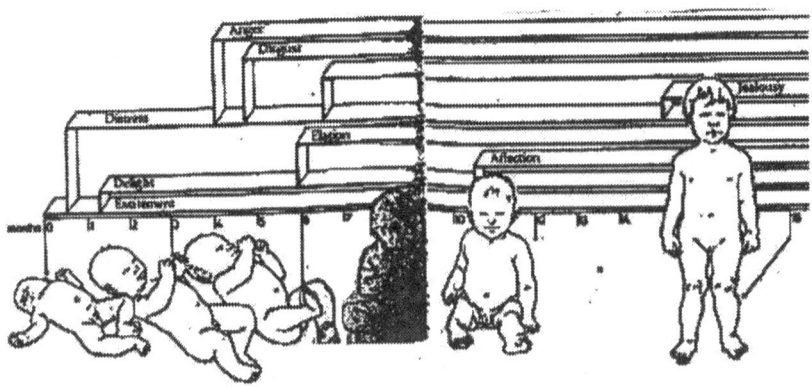

Figure 8-4 Development of Emotion The mature human is able to experience and recognize a wide variety of emotional responses. This capacity is not present at birth, but is developed through pre-maturity by an increased experience of emotional stimuli coinciding with the brain's development. One theory on early emotional development considers that newborn infants originally experience only a generalized sensation of excitement, which soon polarizes into pleasure or distress. As the child matures, these two sensations branch into the more subtle distinctions of the emotions as we know them; the more subtle the distinction between emotions, the later a child experiences them. The Brain: A User's Manual, pp. 230-231

Always, with unconditional love, the goal is independence, then interdependence, rather than dependency. Progress, however, must be gradual and geared to the needs of the child. A woman who herself is emotionally healthy soon learns, both by instinct and observation, to know her own child and to guide his/her development. All caregivers of infants lose the sharp edge of self and other-than-self for a time, fusing with the infant to intuit what the child needs. Many women are afraid to get this close to another for fear of losing their own identity—one possible explanation of why women leave their children to other caretakers. However, a woman and her mate are the child's teachers about love and life. As such, they can foster or weaken the child's foundation for subsequent academic and social achievements.

Psychiatrists, teachers, and historians agree—today's children are different. The transformation of family dynamics and composition has changed the nature of the community, schools, and standards of society. At one time, stability in the lives of children came from a family structure. That structure no longer exists—society no longer supports it. Now, less than 11 percent of families retain the image of a biological father working and a biological mother staying at home.

Two parents in a family make an enormous difference. Too often boys without fathers do not do well in school. Girls without fathers do not know how to relate to a male until they are involved in a sexual relationship during their teen years. Consequently girls may have no guidelines as to what a satisfactory relationship can be.

In the next chapter, we shall examine how fathers and mothers influence their children (sometimes for a lifetime) during these critical early years.

Table 8-A

Influences of Caregiver—Early Development of nervous system (Vaughan)

FUNCTION	PATTERNS AT BIRTH	TIME INTERVAL	CARE NEEDS	IMPORTANCE IN DEVELOPMENT
O X Y G E N	• In utero, the baby uses progressively more oxygen in growth of the brain; at birth, baby is hungry for oxygen as chest has not adjusted for the intake of air • The brain requires twice as much oxygen as other tissues of the body • Early oxygen is a factor in giving life to brain cells, hence closely related to physical and mental health	• Immediately after birth up to 2 months • In first few months of life • In first few moths of life	• The baby should be within mother's reach and observation in order to help with breathing • Holding and fondling is helpful to facilitating breathing • Crying in first few weeks signifies oxygen need; baby should be soothed promptly • Daily fresh air	• The brain needs oxygen and glucose for metabolism • Poor brain metabolism is one factor involved in our response to stress as an adult • The myelin sheath, which protects nerve fibers and improves synaptic transmission, is not developed completely. The myelin sheathing permits nerves to conduct impulses 12 times faster than those without sheathing • Insufficiently developed blood vessels (which deliver oxygen) lead to inadequate irrigation of nerve cells
B R E A T H I N G	• The infant makes the transition from breathing via the placenta to breathing on his own • The lungs are relatively underdeveloped and breathing is rapid and shallow during the first few weeks.	• Respiratory independence is signaled by the initiation of cooing and babbling (2- 5 Months)	• The stimulation of the mother's touch automatically initiates deeper breathing in the infant • Being held and fondled frequently develops reflexes that prime the breathing mechanism until it is under the control of the nervous system	• Outer breathing (respiration) establishes the inner breathing (metabolism) of the nervous system • Timely development of breathing contributes to good speech development

FUNCTION	PATTERNS AT BIRTH	TIME INTERVAL	CARE NEEDS	IMPORTANCE IN DEVELOPMENT
S U C K I N G	• The sucking reflex may be underdeveloped at birth • The sucking need gradually lessens over the course of the first three years of life	• Approximately 6 weeks • Birth to 3 years or more	• At least 50% of babies need guidance and stimulation of the sucking reflex, which is strengthened by the mother's conviction that her baby can succeed • The infant should be given an opportunity to suck on demand for the first few months.	• Releases tension and leads to true body rest and relaxation • Gives improved shape to the moth and teeth and provides blood supply to the facial muscles • Provides means of nutritional intake • Fosters development of speech (intellectual word making) • Facilitates beginning mental development • Affords pleasure and satisfaction • Gives initial sense of security and success • Provides foundation for exploring the shape and concept of the articles placed in the mouth. • Facilitates smiling and kissing, both in terms of physical capability and emotional response
S L E E P	• The infant lacks sufficient development of brain cells, connection nerve fibers and oxygen. Sleep and nutrition contribute equally to their development • The infant needs no less that 16 hours of sleep per day	• First 3-4 Months • Up to 2 years	• Personal attention to baby • Nearness to baby • Attitude of mother • Gentle stimulation and massage	• Lack of nurturing care can cause child to be fearful of losing consciousness (staying awake may be an unconscious means of allaying anxiety over some vague danger) • Stability of the nervous system and balanced body integration area promoted

FUNCTION	PATTERNS AT BIRTH	TIME INTERVAL	CARE NEEDS	IMPORTANCE IN DEVELOPMENT
MOTOR ACTIVITY	• Brain substance, and in particular, the gray matter, is incompletely developed and cells are unfinished • The blood vessels that supply the nervous system are immature • Higher functioning of the brain takes longer to complete.	• Approximately 18 months to 2 years (to develop coordination and locomotive agility)	• The relatively great immaturity of the newborn underscores the mother's need of knowledge of her individual baby's needs and degree of daily development • Such knowledge allows the mother to encourage and appropriately challenges development of motor skills (i.e. stretching, reaching, holding, sitting, climbing, etc)	• Promotes nervous system control • Provides opportunity to learn locomotive and muscle skills • The first relationship of life activates the feelings of the baby and promotes the nervous system to achieve full functional activity, resulting in unique personality development

FUNCTION	PATTERNS AT BIRTH	TIME INTERVAL	CARE NEEDS	IMPORTANCE IN DEVELOPMENT
BREAST FEEDING AND NUTRITION	• Sucking reflex is present • Child's "roots" for breast nipple • Baby will reject breast if he senses any rejection from mother	• Up to 3 years of age depending on circumstances, the attitudes of the mother and the baby	• Only daily hygiene is necessary as nature provides antiseptic cleansing of nipple • Well-fitting brassiere for the mother to preserve breast muscle tone • Willingness on the part of the mother to interrupt her activities to breastfeed on demand until the baby is old enough to eat solid foods	• Facilitates growth of myelin sheathing (see section on oxygen) • First source of pleasure (child takes in a sense of the goodness of the world through the lips) • Provides neurological alternatives to aggressiveness • Influences adult reaction to food and adult IQ • Breast milk is nutritionally superior to formula and even cows' milk. (Designed for human consumption, it is more easily digested) • Energy needed to grow is not diverted into unnecessary digestive activity • Necessitates the direct attention of the mother • Provides immunity to disease for first 6 months of life • Encourages bonding (easy way to develop an intimate relationship as it also influences the hormonal state of the mother) • Increases the infant's sense of self-worth and security • Economical means of providing nutrition • Relaxing to mother (the hormone, prolactin, is released which promotes feeling of motherliness) • Helps to contract the mother's uterus, helping both her and her womb to get back in shape • Encourages baby's sucking reflex which, in turn, promotes growth (see section on sucking)

Chapter 8—Endnotes

1   Mahler, Margaret, *The Psychological Birth of the Human Infant*, Basic Books, Inc., New York, NY, 1973

2   Rosen, Mortimer, M.D. and Rosen, Lynn, EDD., *In the Beginning: Your Baby's Brain Before Birth*, Plume Book, New Amsterdam Library, New York, N.Y., 1975

3   Mahler, op cit

4   Ribble, Margaret A., M.D., *The Rights of infants*, Columbia University Press, New York, N.Y., 1943, 13th printing l957

5   Maguire, Jack and the Philip Leif Group, Inc., *Care and Feeding of the Brain*, Doubleday, New York, NY 1990

6   Meaney, Michael, McGill University, Montreal, Canada reported *Buffalo Evening News*, 7/19/00

7   Maguire, op cit p 12

8   Ibid, p.125

9   Ibid, p.43

10   McEwen, Bruce, Rockefeller Institute, New York, N.Y., 1992, *U.S News and World Report*, 8/8/88

11   Ribble, op cit

12   Hastings, Arthur C. PhD, et al, *Health for the Whole Person*, Bantam Books, New York, Toronto, London, l976

13   Masters, Wm, Johnson, Virginia E., Kolodny, Robert, *Masters & Johnson on Sex and Human Loving*, Little, Brown & Co., Boston/Toronto, 1982/85/86

14   Stein, Sara, *The Body Book*, Workman Publishing, New York, NY 1992

15   Prescott, J.W., "Affectional Bonding for the Prevention of Violent Behavior, Neurobiological, Psychological, and Religious/Spiritual Determinants", In *Violent Behavior, Vol. 1: Assessment and Intervention* (Hertzberg L.J. et al), OMA Publishing Corp., New York, NY, 1990

16   *The Brain, A User's Manual*, The Diagram Group, Berkley Books, New York, NY, 1982

17   The Journal Of Pediatrics, cited in *Vegetarian Times*, August 1991, pp.22,24

18   Giffen, Mary, M.D., with Carol Felsenthal, *A Cry for Help*, Doubleday & Co., Garden City, N.Y. 1983

19   Prescott, op cit, p. 95

[20] Prescott, op cit, p. 119 (Also Cited in Riesen 1975, Struble & Reisen, 1987, and Heath, 1975)

[21] Samuels, Mike, M.D. and Nancy Samuels, *The Well Baby Book*, Summit Books, Simon & Schuster, New York, N.Y., 1979

[22] Giffen, op cit

[23] Franz, Dr. Thomas, SUNYAB, Dean, Counseling Psychology Graduate Division, Conversation 9/21/92

Chapter 9

Who Am I—
The Early Journey Of Self

I trust my family and friends, I value beliefs. I have faith in myself. I appreciate being a girl or a boy and I like the traits that define my masculinity or femininity.[1]

L. Leight, Author

Opening our hearts can mean letting our children make their own mistakes—and learn from them…opening our hearts to our children can mean loving them and ourselves enough to set boundaries that as adults we know they are unprepared to set.-…opening our hearts to our children, with no conditions does not mean we will always say "yes" to what they do. It does mean that we will, to the best of our ability, say "yes" to who they are.[2]

Melissa Galey West

Every child born into this world has a fundamental right to experience the trust in self and others to which Leight refers in the preceding quote. The degree to which each child experiences trust and identity is determined to a large extent by the early relationship offered by the parents, especially the mother. An unbroken sense of trust developed between the mother and father and the infant forms the basis of identity in the child.

A trusting relationship gives rise to a sense of "I" (boy) or "I" (girl) who is lovable. This, in turn, provides the foundation for identity as an adult, from which a sense of inner continuity is derived.

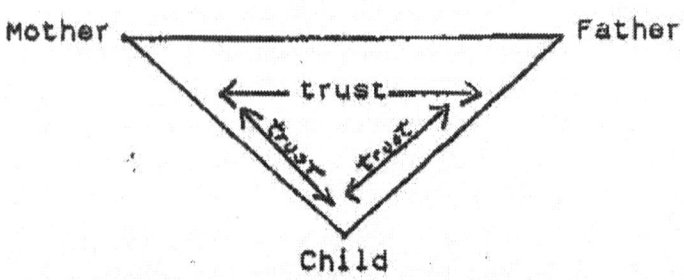

Figure 9-1 Trust Relationship (Straight)

Identity in the adult means a sense of inner continuity and sameness. Our adult identity provides us with the capacity to remain the same person despite changing demands in relationships and life circumstances. Adult individuals who have accomplished a separate, clearly delineated identity can offer themselves more freely to another in a relationship of closeness and separateness. (In Chapter 11, we shall see more clearly the connection between basic infant trust and harmonious adult relationships.) Establishing an identity means developing self-awareness. For the child, establishing an identity consists of eventually assuming a separate existence from the parents, one that is sufficiently free from anxiety, guilt, and parental standards to allow the child to initiate personal relationships freely.[3]

Identity for the infant-through-toddler stage is developed through a growing awareness of self as a separate individual from mother. Such an awareness encompasses three areas. The infant growing into a toddler gradually comes to see self as:

1. worthy and lovable;

2. a separate individual with beginning autonomy;

3. a boy or a girl.

Toddlers accomplish this growth principally by interaction with their parents.

A primitive identity has already been forming on an unconscious level in the womb with the unique first relationship with the mother. The task of parents is to bring such an identity to consciousness free from fear and anxiety. The critical time for such psychic birth is from conception to approximately three years of age. I use the term psychic birth to denote the more gradual development of the less visible psychological and spiritual components of the infant's wholeness and the child's growing awareness of self.

If one has considered the concept of psychic birth at all, one must admit that our awareness of self must have a point of beginning. Most parents believe it begins at birth. However, as the embryo-fetus-infant develops its body parts, there is a concept of self, however primitive, forming in the limbic system and the cerebral cortex of the brain, undifferentiated but responsive (The limbic system, which envelops the top of the brain stem largely controls emotions and behavior, including sex and aggression). We now know that our cells have genetic chemical messages incorporated in them (by means of DNA and RNA) that direct their growth (i.e., specific cells for the eyes, the digestive system, the brain, and the nervous system, etc.) As these systems develop, the infant in the womb begins a primitive sense of being and responds at that level. He or she is developing a unique spirit. The spirit cannot be added on at some distant moment in life. It results from the harmonious interaction right from the beginning of conception of the physical and psychological aspects of being interacting with optimal environmental factors. We cannot, therefore, underestimate the importance of an accepting womb environment to promote that sense of being and unique spirit.

At birth, this primitive sense of self is no longer automatically taken care of. It is abruptly brought into awareness. An "I" has been born who has to cry to signal his/her needs. Before this, every want was supplied automatically in the womb. At this point, the mother becomes even more important in the concept of who the child becomes. These infant feelings and a sense of mutual trust are in the unconscious at the earliest stages of life and before language. They are expressed by the baby's liveliness of response to the mother and visible anxiety upon separation from her. This total body communication is transmitted on a non-verbal level and remains part of the development of the infant's sense of the world. As we shall see in the next chapter, it is the basis on which trust in adulthood is built. In adulthood it is still conveyed to others on an unconscious, non-verbal level.

This unbroken line of trust from the time of mother acceptance in the womb to the achievement of verbal and reciprocal response on the part of the infant cannot be supplied by a caretaker other than the mother. Her body—and then her presence—is the infant's world and can only be separated as the infant's sense of self becomes strong enough to withstand the separation. The physical ability to walk and talk (necessary for separation) takes up to three years. The emotional, intellectual, and spiritual development goes hand-in-hand with that development, inextricably interwoven.

Studies verify that the quality of the relationship is enhanced and strengthened in the time infant and mother spends in eye contact in the first month. Early bonding at the time of delivery and shortly thereafter has been scientifically accepted. Eventually, we will come to document the benefits of continued care by the mother in early years.

Much has been written and studied about bonding. Science now admits to a critical time immediately after birth when the mother and child "bond". It could be better described as a recognition period when the newly displaced infant recognizes the familiar presence in which he has lived for nine months. At the same time, the mother sees for the first time the embodiment of all her fantasies of what the baby in the womb might look like. Actual bonding is only developed over a much longer period of time.

However this early bonding time is very important and hospitals are now encouraging such time for mother and child to be together. LeBoyer has an interesting pause in this procedure where he places the baby in warm water to help it "relax" and then brings it to the mother. He explained at a lecture I attended that this allowed a moment of needed separation for the new identity of the baby to begin while still acknowledging the need to be close to the mother. Such prior relaxation allows even closer bonding. The infant is ready and the mother is waiting.

The process I have been describing is the ideal. It does not say that adopted children cannot mature normally with a good sense of self. It depends on the relationship formed after the adoption. However, the seeking of the biological mother in adult years by those who have experienced adoption, although their family life has been good, indicates to me that some sense of loss was experienced and needs to be laid to rest.

Is s/he lovable? The infant doesn't ask that question specifically. However, if s/he is cared for physically, held and caressed, is stimulated with words and smiles of sincere welcome, s/he senses s/he is OK. Each day of such welcoming care brings a new set of responses from the infant as mother and infant renew their acquaintance on a conscious level.

If the infant is breastfed, a sense of trust and identity is promoted on several different levels. The food is easily digestible, nourishing, sterile, and readily available, allowing the infant's energy to be directed to growth and development, rather than to overcome digestive upsets. Breastfeeding also promotes a sense of closeness, emotional responsiveness, and physical satisfaction as the infant's skin is stimulated and the sucking response is activated.

The mother also benefits from this exchange with her new infant. Using her body's natural abilities, the mother produces both physical and emotional health benefits for herself. Breastfeeding contributes to the health of the uterus after birth. Oxytocin, a hormone secreted to allow the milk to flow more easily into the milk ducts, also helps the uterus to contract, thereby reducing the risk of hemorrhage and restoring the mother's figure to "before baby" size.

Science is now reporting that breastfeeding can be a deterrent to breast cancer as it lessens the time a woman ovulates. There is also scientific acceptance that most breast cancer begins in milk ducts.[4] These are important findings since one in every eight women in the United States will suffer breast cancer at some time during their lives.[5]

Nature cooperates further. When the mother gives birth, her endorphin level (nature's tranquilizer) rises 10 times above the normal level for the benefit of the mother as well as the child. The hormone, prolactin, is provided to the mother to increase her desire to nurture. These physical changes help to provide the mothers with insight and an ability to intuit her baby's feelings—almost a form of telepathy.

Disruption of this interactive identity formation process during the first three years of life, and especially during this period of incorporation, makes the formation of a healthy adult identity more difficult.

As Erikson maintains: "All subsequent development—physical, psychological and spiritual—remains subordinate to and based on this time of the incorporate mode."[6] This is the time when the infant (1) internalizes and takes in nutrition for the body; (2) derives emotional support for psycho-social development; and (3) develops a sense of the meaning of the world. In Chapter 11, we shall see more clearly the connection between basic trust and harmonious adult relationships.

How Trust Answers The Question—Am I Lovable?

Just how does an infant develop a sense of being worthy and lovable? If the infant's needs are met as they arise and growth proceeds as nature intended, a sense of self as good and a sense of control over one's environment is formed in the infant on an unconscious, nonverbal level. This sense of self as good permeates all behavior, fostering a sense of security in the infant obtainable in no other way. It has been said that infants learn of their world first through their lips (linked to 5 cranial nerves). They incorporate the feeling of being OK from the warmth and security of their mother's arms. They take in a sense of acceptance with their mother's milk.

A sense of faith is transmitted to infants in the forming of basic trust. Given the opportunity to give and receive love as they grow, infants develop a sense of Divine Love—a sense of an all embracing goodness of people and the world in general. A sense of gratitude, in a primitive form, is thus elicited at an early age, to be built on in adulthood. A sense of gratitude, says Selye, who first defined the concept of stress, is a source of relieving stress in human beings of any age.

An infant's trust in self and in the integrity of the *other* (at this time, the mother) is basic to building a sense of identity. At birth, the infant's self and mother are blended into one, and self can only become a separate entity as the infant grows physically and develops the brain and neurological system in an accepting environment. The mother, in turn, develops a new appreciation of herself and a sense of accomplishment as she watches her baby's peaceful and tranquil growth. She relaxes with her infant, and the mutuality of their feelings is extremely important as the first experience of "friendly otherness."

Erikson maintains that the establishment of enduring patterns for the resolution of basic trust-versus-mistrust in an individual is the task of the ego, and thus is initially a task for maternal care.

> The amount of trust derived from earliest infantile experience does not seem to depend on absolute quantities of food or demonstrations of love, but rather on the quality of the maternal relationship. Mothers create a sense of trust in their children by that kind of administration which in its quality combines sensitive care of the baby's individual needs and a firm sense of personal trustworthiness within the trusted framework of their culture's lifestyle. This forms the basis in the child for a sense of identity which will later combine a sense of being "all right", of being oneself, and of becoming what other people trust one will become.[7]

In other words, a mother who is a mature woman, already grounded in her choice of life-styles and who has a warm, welcoming attitude, as well as the knowledge of how to care for her infant, provides an optimal environment for infant identity development.

Dr. Mike Samuels and his wife broaden this early influence on the infant to the relationship with parents. At the time of birth, a new era is entered into by both parents and infant. Samuels describes the shock of birth as a gift that allows parents to let go of old ways and patterns and to permit "instinct and deep emotions to guide behavior." Samuels points out that the synchronous afterbirth dance of mother and child, by which they gain each other's attention, holds much more learning for both than an observer can see. What appears to be just excitement on the part of a one-day-old infant is revealed by slow motion analysis, to be purposeful movement—movement that is in "precise shared rhythm with adult speech pattern[s]…mirroring the linguistic forms of adults; [indeed] babies are building into their bodies the rhythms and nuances of language months before they learn to speak themselves".[8]

Simultaneously, in the performance of this synchronous dance, the baby learns to trust. Trust is as equally important as the development of language in this critical time period. Speech is not developed in a vacuum. Trust is the environment in which language can develop. The mutual relaxation of the mother and baby and their mutual sense of belonging and acceptance benefits both. The profound bonding that occurs not only promotes the infant's development. It also evokes in the mother appropriate maternal behavior. Physically abetted by hormones, especially when the mother is breastfeeding, mother and infant are off to a good start of parallel growth.

The early critical period we have referred to above is often technically known as the oral-respiratory-sensory stage, when the organs used in sucking and breathing are being developed. Details of this stage are provided in the preceding chapter. However, it is also important to recognize that this is also a period when all sense organs, including the skin, are receptive and hungry for proper stimulation. If such stimulation is available and received by the infant in the critical early months, then other organs and modes of behavior develop in the right order (i.e., digestion, elimination, and genitalia). A trusting infant, secure in the sense that s/he is cared for and important to someone, matures as nature intended. General good health is preceded and directed by a sense of well-being. In the mother-infant exchange of giving and receiving, the child learns to receive and accept what is given—a first step in learning social skills. This new being, finding its way in the world, learns this social modality as it learns to regulate its organ system. Surely, it is easy to see that they both influence one another and are influenced by the type of care given and received. For example, gentle cuddling helps the chest muscles to relax and thus promotes the breathing process and development of the lungs.

In other words, it is as though nature is putting a priority on the loving relationship of mother and child so that maturation can proceed in an orderly manner.

Experienced doctors who have observed many infants have noted that the ability to love is not a separate reaction that appears automatically at a certain period in the child's life. Instead, it is a highly complicated pattern of behavior that begins in the womb, is fostered physically at birth when the first hunger pangs are appeased by the mother, and is further developed psychologically in response to the mother's presence and care.

At birth, mother and child are psychologically one, with the exception of the unconscious, which has developed certain primitive impressions and nuances in the womb. Separated physically at birth, their intimate dance with each other gives both mother and child a sense of intense satisfaction and rightness. As the infant expresses its individual needs and mother meets those needs, a pattern of personality emerges. If the little one's needs are met with love and oral satisfaction, s/he incorporates a sense of trust and control of the world. This sense of control is primary to reducing the infant's helplessness and is the beginning of separation and autonomy. "I am an individual different from my mother and I have control over my environment." As proper stimulation is presented at appropriate times, this sense of being grows. The process of separation and autonomy is not completed, however, until about the third year of life. As the child gains greater motor control and a concurrent ability to see, hear, eat, sit, walk, grasp toys, and distinguish voices and people, a greater sense of autonomy is fostered. "Look Ma, no hands" is the attitude that begins to develop.

The amount of trust a child incorporates is directly related to the degree of trust the mother experiences with her spouse. It is parents who develop trust in their child—not only the mother. If the parents are too immature to trust, it is difficult to convey such a sense to the infant.

All parents have some sense of not being able to measure up—especially with their first child. It is a period of enormous change and a sense of not being able to cope is natural and universal. Confidence in one's self, reassurance from one's spouse, information, and experience soon allay this type of anxiety.

Trust on the part of infants means that they expect with confidence that their needs will be satisfied. If the child is hungry and is fed with a digestible substance to a full measure of satisfaction in an ambiance of acceptance, his or her expectation (hope) of someone being there to meet his/her need is also met, and a sense of being important to someone is initiated. If this process is repeated daily, to the same level of satisfaction by a competent mother, who has been familiar to the infant from the beginning of life in the womb, it is easy to see how the beginning of ego identity and trust is formed. "I am someone and I have the power to get my needs met." Thus confidence builds, in self and in *other* through a nonverbal exchange of love.

To terminate or diminish this budding relationship and newly forming sense of identity for both mother and child within four months—the legal amount of leave allowed the working mother—has several potential risks. It can disrupt the process of the formation of trust, identity, and autonomy; it can delay or, perhaps, prevent the completion of the nervous system; and it can deprive a child of the right to develop his or her sense of maleness or femaleness at a critical time.

When this loving exchange is ended abruptly, there is a sense of loss, both for the infant and the mother. Confusion, anxiety, and mistrust enter the infant's experience of the world. Some infants respond with rage and anger. Others experience a sense of sadness and alienation. Spiritually, the infant unconsciously makes meaning of the separation, interpreting it, albeit on a primitive level, as a rejection or loss. Physically, such a separation may give rise to susceptibility to irritability, digestive upsets, and allergies in the infant. Moreover, lack of trust development at this critical time may hamper the full expression of adult sexuality. (see Chapter 11)

To summarize, the infant, newly deprived at birth of the security experienced while in the mother's body, seeks comfort through the incorporation of the mother's milk, body warmth, and her accepting love and security. At the same time, infants are incorporating into their psyches a sense of trust. Their ego begins to develop. As ego and trust develop, the child's sense of autonomy and self, separate from mother, begin to grow.

A sense of separate self is very important in adult mental health. Acceptance of the concept that ultimately we are alone in our journey through life comes with a healthy ego and a successful struggle against anxiety, which is endemic in our society. The most accepted theory of anxiety holds that anxiety derives from a fear of separation. Thus, it behooves us, as parents, to deal very carefully with the separation of mother and child in the first stages of life. All children need the certainty that the caregiver will not abandon them.

To illustrate the effects of too early separation, let us consider the case of Gregory, the second child of a loving couple. Gregory's mother was extremely ill after birthing. On the doctor's advice, the infant was placed with a foster couple for several months until the mother's health improved. (The doctor reasoned that the baby's cries would distress the mother and impede her recovery since she could not respond to the child as she normally would.) The child received quite adequate care from the foster parents. He was clothed, fed, and kept clean. However, when three months later Gregory returned to his parents, he resembled a severely malnourished child. He had not eaten well and his sleep was restless. He had been grieving for the loss of his familiar environment—his mother. He had been physically nourished, but had not received that unconditional, familiar love that is so necessary for infant well-being. Gregory was quickly restored to a normal appearance and nutritional status in the presence of the love of his parents and siblings.

What was not so easily restored, and was not apparent at the time, was that Gregory had not been able to develop that sense of trust and ego identity on the unconscious level of an infant that is so fundamental to healthy adult integration.

He had been separated from his mother at a critical time for the development of trust and identity and unfortunately could not reclaim that time.

Gregory developed physically and intellectually in a normal fashion, but was not successful with relationships. Even to his siblings, he appeared different in an undefined way. He was a gentle fellow, always seeking affection and love. Without having developed appropriate boundaries, his seeking took the abnormal path of sexual abuse of a sibling. Finally, after insurmountable difficulties at school, he underwent a period of treatment in a mental hospital. His adjustment to adult life was clearly below his true or innate capacity to develop.

None of his siblings showed any such pathology, and they became successful adults. Although Gregory had had the same parents and experienced the same accepting family environment, he had never been able to form a "clear identity." He lacked a sense of self-worth and so sought infantile nurturance in the guise of adult sexuality, unable as he was to form relationships with others as an equal. He never overcame the loss of interaction with his mother at the critical time immediately following birth.

Gregory's case helps us to realize that learning to trust is not an intellectual exercise. It is the result of organically experiencing, at a critical time, a trusting relationship without barriers or conditions. Individuals must develop trust in at least one other human being in order to know themselves as either a male or female being of the human species and to know that they have self-worth. Varying degrees of trust formed in infancy result in varying degrees of trust in adulthood.

A sense of unconscious trust in the womb is directed from the infant to the accepting mother. Doesn't it make sense that, after birth, that same *other* is the focus of the infant in bringing that instinctive sense of trust into conscious awareness? Mother and child are inextricably linked at the time of birth, each creating feelings in the other. As Erikson states: "All feelings are initiated in the oneness between the young infant and its mother in which feelings of recognition, acceptance and tenderness are exchanged unconditionally through looks, caresses and words."[9]

This is the period we first learn about love, about giving and receiving, and about commitment. These same feelings stay with us throughout life. Mental health professionals can testify to serving many clients who have not experienced these early feelings adequately and who, as a result, are handicapped as adults in expressing or experiencing their feelings.

If I Can Trust, I Know I Can Function

The second component of identity formation is a sense of autonomy. Autonomy is the power to exercise one's will freely and responsibly. Obviously, a child from birth to three years cannot have total autonomy. However, this period is when the foundation for adult achievement and use of free will is laid. It is the beginning of ego development, the primary function of which is to direct a person so that his or her needs may be fulfilled in the world. Lack of such a foundation for autonomy, or weak ego development, makes it more difficult for the adult to be free and autonomous. The development of autonomy requires the gradual unfolding of dependence toward independence that is a component of good parenting for any child. Parent actions that contribute to autonomy include the following:

1. Providing appropriate stimulation for good motor control

2. Offering healthy nutrition at appropriate times for good digestion

3. Modeling and encouraging good eating habits (not to be confused with neat eating habits)

4. When breastfeeding, weaning the child gradually according to the child's readiness and timeframe, not the mother's convenience

5. Allowing the child to do as much as possible for himself or herself while providing support and affirmation

6. Accepting the child's own level and speed of maturation, without comparing it to a neighbor's child or another sibling

7. Affirming the child in all the areas of the parent-child relationship

8. Providing firm limits on behavior and protection from danger.

If these guidelines are observed, each new accomplishment, then, will maintain and foster the child's confidence and develop his or her ego.

Jack Dominion, psychiatrist and author, stresses the importance of affirmation in the formation of autonomy. He writes:

> For no one should enter this world as a beggar. The helpless child has a right to feel that life is not a concession granted to it by kind permission of its parents. It has a claim to independence and value and it can only learn by the way it feels it is treated.... This sense of autonomy exhibits itself from the very moment of birth when the physical separation establishes the beginning of two models, the world of "me" and the world of "not me." For too often this early world has been

constructed and experienced as the world of the permissible and the forbidden. Development largely dependent on authoritarian principles has left many people with a sense only of that which is permissible or forbidden. Affirmation, in fact, aims to stress the enlarging acquisition of separate existence and achievement such as standing, walking, putting sentences together…encouraging their development with just the right amount of help and giving credit for the achievement where it belongs.

Dominion further asserts that affirmation:

> is not only facilitation of achievement, [but] even more important it is the imparting of the sense that the achievement rightly belongs to the source of origin [the child]. Affirmation is achievement by an enlargement of self and a reduction of infantile dependence.[10]

Brian, almost three years of age, was a very agile child who had perfected the art of running. He would run up and down the driveway repeatedly, exhibiting his agility and power. After each run, he would wait to be told, "That was great, Brian. You are a wonderful runner." The running was a satisfaction in itself, but his sense of self was enhanced by having his ability recognized verbally (verbal affirmation), and he would wait each time for recognition of his prowess. Affirmation was as important to him as the power to run.

There are many other ways to affirm another person, some of which are more subtle—looks, body posture, and a genuine appreciation of the other. The need for affirmation begins in the womb and continues from birth to the end of life in varying degrees. Because of the authoritarian system by which we live, in which conformity and obedience are valued, we as parents are apt to forget that a feeling of goodness rests largely on the affirmation of the child's feeling, thought, word or actions. Affirmation ensures children that their sense of badness is not larger than their sense of goodness, or that their inappropriate actions have not threatened their personal significance in the eyes of those who matter most to them.

One example of an authoritarian attitude is the reaction of the mother of six fully grown children. Upon learning that the nervous system did not mature until approximately eighteen months after birth, she quickly responded, "That's a good reason to control the child, since he won't be able to control himself." Infants in early months do not need punishment or control to grow, only love, order, and affirmation. However, it is important to note this must be genuine and not excessive. Praise that is insincere is likely to make the child feel insecure. Table 9-1 at the end of the chapter illustrates the difference between praise and encouragement.

To develop autonomy, the child requires a firmly developed sense of early trust that is convincingly continued. Growing infants and toddlers must feel that the choices they make, which are often attributed to mischief or misbehavior, will not jeopardize their trust in self and others.

Maria Montessori, a doctor and educator, also underscores the importance of autonomy, but states it in more spiritual terms:

> The newborn child should be seen as a "spiritual embryo", a spirit enclosed in flesh in order to come into the world…. The child possesses a psychic life…a hidden, imprisoned spirit is born and grows, animating little by little the passive flesh, calling forth the voice of the will, coming into the light of consciousness with the force of a living creature being born into the world. But in the new environment another being of enormous power awaits it and ultimately dominates it…. The child…must come to live for itself in the environment. Like the physical embryo, the spiritual embryo must be protected by an external environment animated by the warmth of love and the richness of value, where it is wholly accepted and never inhibited…. The inner effort of the child must remain sacred.[11]

Many psychologists agree with Montessori, but they express their findings in terms of ego. William Glasser is known for his reality theory.[12] He defines ego as the core of identity formation. At full development, the ego includes the functions of intellect, emotions and the individual's unique pattern of reacting, called personality. The ego directs individuals so that they may fulfill their needs in the world, while protecting themselves from danger. Glasser finds: "In the infant it is easily seen that 'the world' is his treatment at the hands of his caretaker." If the caretaker is able to meet the needs of the infant, the ego of the infant grows. The dangers of the world are commensurate with the development of a person's ability to cope. The loving caretaker withdraws support only when the infant develops to the degree necessary to cope on his or her own.

In the following diagram, Panel I depicts the fact that the ego of the infant and mother cannot be totally separated initially. In Panel II, if the ego is properly nourished, the necessary physical growth maturation will be completed, the child will be able to cope, and the separation process will be initiated. In the adult stage (Panel III), the ego is able to deal with reality (the world), separate from parents.

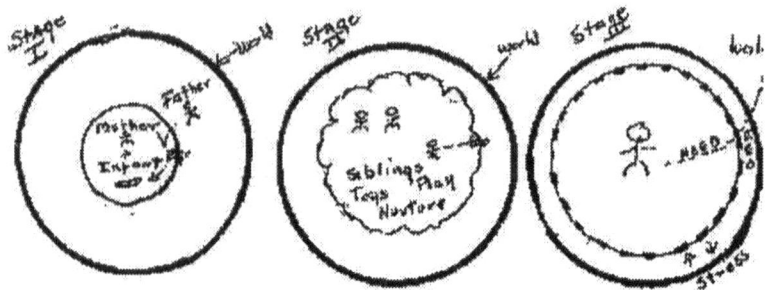

Figure 9-2 Separation Illustration (adapted from Glasser)

The ego develops a variety of reactions that can be classed under the heading of emotion. Although emotions are primarily psychological, they also have a bearing on physical feelings. Good emotions bring about a sense of physical well-being, muscular relaxation or a pleasant degree of tension. Good emotions elicit feelings of warmth, strength, and physical confidence in our body and our ability to function.

By contrast, unpleasant emotions may be accompanied by tense muscles, digestive upsets, and many other physical complaints. Our bodies feel generally weak and we lack confidence. Often psychosomatic diseases result. Poor ego development means a person is lacking in positive emotion because of poor functioning. Life is difficult and the ego often chooses unpleasant emotional reactions and behaviors.

Studies of anxiety in children have demonstrated that those who are free of inordinate anxiety come from homes where the family is relaxed and friendly and the children are loved and disciplined. According to author June Callwood, over-punished and underadmired children test highest in anxiety:

> Anxiety prevents the development of genuine love and interferes with the sex drive. A tense father and mother are as contagious as Typhoid Mary. Anxiety about money is often conditioned by parents who discuss financial problems in a worried manner. Even an infant can sense his parent's anxieties and incorporate them.[13]

We need to be conscious of the effect our attitudes and behavior have on even the youngest infant.

Beginning Core Gender Identity

In the beginning of this chapter, we stated that the third requisite for identity formation is that the infant growing into a toddler gradually comes to see self as a boy or a girl. How often have you heard a two and one-half year old exclaim heatedly and very definitively, "I am a girl" or "I am a boy." The emotion that accompanies this declaration evidences the learning and development going on internally within the child.

Sherman Silber, in his book *The Male* states,

> The scientific evidence is that sexual identity and sexual preferences are determined during the first two years of life and thus would appear to be innate by the time anybody pays attention to them. But they are not innate. They are determined by the social environment to which the child is exposed in the earliest months of life.[14]

The reader must bear in mind that infants bring to their social environment a unique physical and hormonal makeup that will also influence their response to the environment and thus influence their sexual identity. Together with the development of the senses, motor ability, and personality, infants gradually begin the process of identifying with the parent of the same sex. They observe both parents, their sameness and their differences. They begin to notice how similar they are to one parent. If both parents are loving and involved with care of the child, the task is made easier. If one or the other or both are unkind, abusive, or neglectful, the choice becomes complex.

Silber describes the process:

> The child assimilates in his brain all of the different behaviors of the father figure and the mother figure in his life, just as the immigrant child assimilates the two different languages that his ears are constantly bombarded with. In accordance with whether he is reared as male or as female, he will code the behavior of the like sex parent as positive and the opposite sex parent as negative. Father and Mother may have remarkably similar attitudes and liberated views of their responsibility toward society. The important thing is for the infant male to perceive that the male cues that surround him are positive and that the female cues complement those cues.[15]

When Jeff was about two, when asked, would playfully alternate between saying he was a girl or a boy. However, Jeff was almost three when this exchange with his mother occurred while I was present. It had been a little family joke to say to

Jeff, "You are full of pfefferneuse." Jeff and his mother were playfully hugging when his mother, as she had many times before, laughingly asked, "Jeff are you full of pfefferneuse?" Jeff laughed and grunted. Again his mother said, "Jeff are you full of pfefferneuse?" And Jeff, now preoccupied with one of his toys, said "No, only girls are full of pfefferneuse." His mother, surprised at the new response said, "Jeff, why are girls full of pfefferneuse?" He said very factually, "that's where they get their strength from." More surprised than ever, mother persisted, "If you are not a girl, where do you get your strength from?" Instantly Jeff replied, still absorbed in his play, "I have a penis—and that makes me strong!" A 6-month change of attitude!

In many ways beyond our conscious knowledge, we treat little boys and girls differently. This seems to be universal and cannot be hidden. Potter has produced a film called *The Touch Film*[16] which does a wonderful job of explaining some of these differences. Learning theorists have deplored this different treatment as a basis of inequality between the sexes. However, nature intended parents to influence their children in a complementary fashion according to their sex. Their principal task together is to teach children how to love. They do this principally by example. It is important that they do so as model examples of male and female. The parent's love for each other has a positive effect on the infant and helps him/her to form an identity as a boy or girl. When the child observes the loving interaction between mother and father, the child will view them as different and will automatically program himself or herself according to the parent of the same sex. Discordant messages confuse this straightforward identification and, in later adulthood, encumber the working out of a whole identity as male or female.

The identification process is a very gradual one, starting with the mother. If that relationship is satisfactory and furthers the growth of the infant, he or she can then proceed with the selection of traits s/he wishes to emulate or which feel right to his/her individual growth pattern.

In the newborn, this process is unconscious and proceeds according to his gene/hormonal pattern. If relationships do not proceed satisfactorily, the identification/selection process is impaired by unsatisfied emotional needs and therefore cannot be decisive. By approximately age three, the inner knowledge developed by the child that he is a boy or she is a girl is generally known as core gender identity.

John Money, well-known researcher in core gender identity, compares the identification process to the development of language. The age of establishing conceptual language is also the age of establishing a self-concept. This self-concept is by its very nature gender-differentiated. It is often referred to as the core gender identity (Stoller, 1968).

Establishment of core gender identity is obviously a process of learning, insofar as it takes place in social interaction. Establishment of language also is a process of learning. But the establishment of…speech is possible only in the human species; it first requires a brain that has been programmed to be able to acquire speech. Then it requires that this brain interact with other members of the species who have a history of using a language. This interaction…is programmed to take place at a specific and sensitive period in the juvenile life cycle, if it is to be optimally effective. Then the establishment of language is remarkably rapid, and above all, remarkably ineradicable…. On the basis of today's evidence— and here one must be judiciously tentative—it appears that the period of greatest risk for errors of gender-identity formation, of long-lasting effect in the brain, is after birth, and at around the time of acquiring the native language.

Gender identity differentiation of the brain after birth is a process that one may surmise to resemble differentiation of the internal rather than the external genitalia. Neither the male nor the female system is totally and completely obliterated, but one becomes dominant over the other. A boy knows how to do and say boy things, because he simultaneously recognizes girl things as unfitting for him to express, though requiring complementary or reciprocity of reaction on his part—and vice versa for girls…. The more one stops to think about it, the more remarkable does it seem that an infant brain can receive the sound waves of two languages spoken around him, and differentiate them as two non-overlapping systems, vocally and linguistically. The task is facilitated if each language is spoken by different people. Then each language can be identified as belonging to the person or persons speaking it. There is less confusion than when the same speaker alternates between two languages. The parallel with gender identity formation is obvious, for the masculine and feminine models in a child's environment are usually quite clearly differentiated, regardless of the amount of overlap that may be culturally permitted.[17]

This unconscious process, described so well by Money, is worked out more and more consciously as the child grows to adulthood with the maturing of reasoning powers and the development of emotional control. With maturity, each individual more freely experiences his or her own gender and is secure in that identity.

As the child forms a more positive identification with one or the other parent, s/he also chooses traits from each parent—some from the same sex parent, others from the parent of the opposite sex—gradually forming a unique personality.

Picture the complications that could ensue if say Bobby dislikes his father or feels rejected or resented by his mother. He may have a hard time understanding what a boy should be. Again, anxiety clouds the sense of self as a particular gender. Dr. Silber, quoted previously asserts strongly:

> If in the earlier years of life a little boy becomes fixed on an image of himself that is confusing, then he may grow up as out of step with society as a child who is born in a house where no language is spoken or where the language of the country in which he lives is forbidden.[18]

To summarize; basic trust, autonomy, a sense of self as lovable, and a sexual identity as either masculine or feminine are formed from approximately zero to three years of age. Parental love and attention during these years, especially on the part of the mother, is a function of this formation (Table 9-1).

This period of basic trust development and identity formation is also a period when children learn how to view their body and body parts. The cues that children receive in their early months and years of life will be subtle, numerous, and complex. They can be difficult to change. Most often, children notice the difference in gender genitalia and toileting. If questions are answered truthfully and easily, the child accepts the explanations as reality and part of the world that is being explored. If shame or uneasiness is exhibited by the parents, the child senses the emotion, while not understanding it, cannot accept the parent's explanation unequivocally, and becomes anxious.

At this particular time, children will find sensual pleasure in examining their genitalia. If parents do not recognize this as normal development, the child will retain a sense of anxiety about pleasure in this area. Of course, the pleasure derived by the child has no relation to the adult goal of intercourse or adult sexual pleasure, but parents with their greater knowledge and, perhaps, faulty training may interpret this normal part of growth and development as perverted and shame the youngster.

Scientific researchers have detected erect penises and orgasms even in the womb.

Children mature in the erotic area of their sexuality in varying degrees, as with walking, talking, and other developmental milestones. Parents have to be guided by their own child, as well as by their own intuition and knowledge. What is most important is to maintain open communication, offer factual information, and express love for the child openly and often. To do otherwise is to make the pathway to mature adult sexuality difficult.

It should be noted that too little or inconsistent mothering of the infant can result in precocious sexual development. Under ideal conditions in which parents are emotionally well adapted and the baby is wanted and loved, the sex impulses of the child do not necessarily become a problem until near adolescence, although they are definitely in evidence. When emotional hunger of the child is not satisfied, or when the early emotional relationship with the mother is overdeveloped because of insecurity in the mother, sex habits or erotic activities…inevitably become exaggerated. The unmothered child will stimulate himself…which has a direct bearing on early infantile masturbation. In turn, premature…stimulation of the sex organs brings about fatigue and a sense of uneasiness in the child and anxiety in the parent…. Almost unknowingly…a conflict is started between the child and his environment which may last throughout his life.[19]

Although the parent's method of dealing with the physical aspects of the sexual development of the child is important at this stage, far more important is the relationship of each parent to the other in the establishment of boy/girl identity. It is primary. In the next chapter, we shall examine the special role of the father.

In brief…

❖ Psychological and spiritual components of the newborn begin at conception with the first cell which is coded for development of the whole person.

❖ Psychic birth, or individuation, is a more gradual process than physical birth.

❖ The child begins the identity process from approximately zero to three years.

❖ The identity process is progressing normally when the child learns in a deep internal sense, by approximately the age of three, that s/he is lovable, s/he has autonomy appropriate to his/her age, and a core gender identity is established.

Table 9-A

• Differences between Praise and Encouragement

- External   • Internal

• Praise   • Encouragement

• Underlying Characteristics	• Message sent to child	• Possible Results	• Underlying Characteristics	• Message sent to child	• Possible Results
• 1. Focus is on external control	"You are worthwhile only when you do what I want." "You cannot and should not be trusted"	• Child learns to measure worth by ability to conform; or, child rebels (views any form of cooperation as giving in)	• Focus is on child's ability to manage life constructively	"I trust you to become responsible and independent"	• Child learns courage to be imperfect and willingness to learn. Child gaining self-confidence and comes to feel responsible for own behavior.
• 2. Focus is on external evaluation	"To be worthwhile you must please me" "Please or perish"	• Child learns to measure worth on how well he/she pleases others. Child learns to fear disapproval.	• Focus is on internal evaluation	"How you feel about yourself and your own efforts is most important."	• Child learns to evaluate own progress and to make own decisions.
• 3. Is rewarded only for well-done completed tasks	"To be worthwhile you must meet my standards"	• Child develops unrealistic standards and learns to measure worth by how closely she/he reaches perfection. Child learns to dread failure.	• Recognizes effort and improvement	"You don't have to be perfect. Effort and improvement are important."	• Child learns to accept efforts of self and others. Child develops desire to stay with tasks (persistence).
• 4. Focuses on self-satisfaction and personal gain	"You're the best. You must remain superior to others to be worthwhile"	• Child learns to be over competitive, to get ahead at the expense of others. Feels worthwhile only when "on ice".	• Focuses on assets, contributions, and appreciation.	"Your contribution counts. We function better with you. We appreciate what you have done."	• Child learns to use talents and efforts for good of all, not only for personal gain. Child learns to feel glad for successes of others as well as for own successes.

Table 9-A—from Hitz R., Driscoll A., "Praise or Encouragement New Insights into Praise: Implications for Early Childhood Teachers" Young Children, July 1988

Table 9-B
The Healthy Personality

First Stage (Almost First Year)	BASIC TRUST	Earlier Form of Autonomy	Earlier Form OF Initiative
Second STAGE (About Second and Third Years)	Later Form of Basic Trust	AUTONOMY	Earlier form Of Initiative
Third Stage (Almost Fourth and Fifth years)	Later Form Of Basic Trust	Later Form of Autonomy	INITIATIVE

Table 9-B The Healthy Personality, Adapted From Erikson, <u>Identity and the Life Cycle</u>

Whenever we try to understand growth, it is well to remember the epigenetic principle which is derived from the growth of organisms in utero. Somewhat generalized, this principle states that anything that grows has a ground plan, and that out of this ground plan the parts arise, each part having its time of special ascendancy, until all parts have arisen to form a functioning whole. At birth the baby leaves the chemical exchange of the womb for the social exchange system of his society, where his gradually increasing capacities meet the opportunities and limitations of his culture. How the maturing organism continues to unfold, not by developing new organs, but by a prescribed sequence of locomotor, sensory and social capacities, is described in child development literature.... It is important to realize that in the sequence of his most personal experiences the healthy child, given a reasonable amount of guidance, can be trusted to obey inner laws of development, laws which create a succession of potentialities for significant interaction with those who tend him. While such interaction varies from culture to culture, it must remain within the proper rate and the proper sequence which govern the growth of a personality as well as that of an organism. Personality can be said to develop according to steps predetermined in the human organism's readiness to be driven toward, to be aware of, and to interact with, a widening social radius, beginning with the dim image of mother and ending with...that segment of mankind which counts in the particular individual's life.[20]

Chapter 9—Endnotes

1 Leight, Lynn, *Raising Sexually Healthy Children*, Rawson Associates, New York, N.Y., 1988

2 West, Melissa Gayle, *If Only I were a Better Mother*, Stillpoint Publishing, Walpole, N.H. 1992

3 Dominion, Jack, *Affirming the Human Personality*, Darton, Longman & Todd, Ltd, London, 1975

4 The Lancet Medical Journal, reported in *Daily Gazette*, 4/27/01

5 Fachelmann, Kathy A., "Motherhood and Cancer", *Science News*, Vol. 142, p.298, October 31, 1992

6 Erikson, Erik, *Identity and the Life Cycle*, W.W. Norton & Co., New York, N.Y., 1959, 1980

7 Ibid, p. 149

8 Samuels, Mike, M.D. and Mary Samuels, *The Well Baby Book*, Summit Books, Simon & Schuster, New York, N.Y., 1979

9 Erikson, op cit

10 Dominion, op cit, p. 158

11 Montessori, Maria, *The Child in the Family*, Translated by Nancy Rockmore Cirillo, Henry Regenery Co., Chicago, Ill., 1970

12 Glasser, William, M.D., "The Ego, Your Bridge to the World", from "Blueprint for Health", *Blue Cross Association*, Vol 20, No. 3, Chicago, Ill, 1960

13 Callwood, June, *Emotions, What They Are and How They Affect Us*, Doubleday & Co., New York, N.Y., 1986

14 Silber, Sherman, J., *The Male from Infancy to Old Age*, Charles Scribner, Inc., New York, N. Y., 1981

15 Ibid

16 Potter, Dr. Jesse, *The Touch Film*, Sterling Products, 500 N. Dearborn St., Chicago, Ill.

17 Money, John, *Man, Woman, Boy, Girl*, John Hopkins University Press, Baltimore, Md., 1973

18 Silber, op cit

19 Ribble, Margaret, M.D., *The Rights of Infants*, Columbia University Press, New York, N.Y., 1957, 1980

20 Erikson, op cit

Chapter 10

Fathers

It may well be that in order to improve the quality of mothering one of the most important things we can do is to encourage boys and men to be good fathers.[1]

Myriam Medzian,

However fundamental women's maternity may be, it is almost nothing in comparison with her spiritual fertility. Woman brings fullness of being, sensibility, and self-revelation to the man who has loved her.[2]

Teilhard de Chardin,

Anthropology, sociology and psychology can show us how we self-limit and give social definition to the gender, how we form and deform. But it can never reduce the pre-conscious personal duality of the sexes to an adequate explanation.[3]

Sam Keen

It was my first inclination to add information about the role of fathers in the preceding chapter. My reasoning was that any discussion on the development of identity must include the influence of the father. Society often fails to recognize or support the extremely important part fathers play in the formation of the sexual identity of both boys and girls. On reviewing my notes, however, it was clear that a separate chapter was needed to present such significant information. The present picture is negative in the extreme.

In 1960, men between the ages of 20 and 49 spent an average of 12.3 years living in families with their minor children. By 1980 that figure had fallen to 7 years. Only one child in three who live outside their fathers' home receive financial support from dad. One-quarter of America's children live in fatherless homes and one-half of those fall below the poverty level.

Ten years after their parents divorce, half the children of the divorced parents had not seen their non-custodial father in a year and one-sixth had seen him once or twice. Fathers have been described as absentee cash registers with visitation rights. There is an increasingly popular view that the courts are prejudiced against dads via restraining orders and welfare regulations.

In the extreme is the fact that at least 3000 fatherless babies are produced each year through artificial insemination. Anonymous sperm donors are gaining in acceptance, further devaluating fatherhood.[4]

Children need fathers! Both boys and girls benefit greatly in their sexual development by a good relationship with their father. Science tells us why and how. Research confirms what experience is teaching us—the vital importance of fathers. But you don't need scientific research—just ask any child!

Keen's statement on the pre-conscious personal duality of the sexes that begins this chapter expresses succinctly my view of the development of masculinity and femininity. As outlined in previous chapters, in the womb, the sexual anatomy of the embryo is influenced by both testosterone and estrogen. In boys, the masculine hormone testosterone acts at a critical time on the previously undefined fetus to produce changes that result in the development of a male infant. However, as Money states: "In normal development, neither the male or the female system is totally and completely obliterated, but one becomes dominant over the other."[5]

Therefore, our sexuality—whether predominantly male or female—has components of both sexes (Keen's duality of the sexes). A psychological sense of being primarily masculine or feminine is built upon this sexual anatomy and hormonal distribution, as well as on the masculine and feminine models presented by mother and father. Both parents contribute to a boy's sense of being masculine and a girl's sense of being feminine. To what degree sexual identity is developed— and whether this development is successfully completed depends in great measure on society's definition of sex roles and the individual parent's response to them.

Although often confused, sex roles and sexual identity are not interchangeable concepts. Kirkpatrick maintains that sexual identity runs deeper and is less conscious than sex-role preference. He defines sexual identity as

> ...an inner conviction about which sex one does in fact belong—a basic commitment with one's maleness and femaleness.... [By contrast] sex role preferences refer to a more conscious desire to play the part which society assigns to one sex or the other.[6]

Thus we see a common, dual thread running through human development from the womb. All human beings are formed by the contribution of one sex cell derived from a male and a female. All embryos, in normal development, receive both estrogen and testosterone but in different amounts. All children have a mother and a father—a masculine and a feminine influence. All human beings retain as part of their make-up not only a biological basis for, but also a psychological sense of, masculinity and femininity in varying degrees. All beings play a role in the sexual culture of their society.

It is when all stages and facets of development (e.g., those related to chromosomes, hormones, parental care, and social conditioning) are coordinated as nature intended that a mature man or woman emerges. Conversely, when one of these stages or facets is imperfectly developed, an immature or incomplete human being results.

Fathers And Mothers: Partners In Healthy Identity And Development

The role of the father is inextricably bound to the role of the mother in the development of the child. As stated previously, the sexes are complementary—equal, but complementary. Father and mother each make a distinctive and indispensable contribution to the unique personality of both boys and girls. The father's indispensability extends far beyond the recreational pleasures he can give his child or the biological heritage he transmits with his sperm.

Often, the importance of the father is measured by his level of involvement in the care of the child. Sharing mealtimes together; participating in bathtime and play activities, a hobby, or outdoor activities; visiting Dad's workplace, or a restaurant (just Dad and me!) or even reading the comics together. These are all wonderful ways a father can show interest in his child while sharing the responsibilities so often viewed inaccurately as the mother's. These activities all serve to help the child bond to his father. However, in addition to these practical means of fathering, there are less visible but equally (or more) important aspects of the presence of the father.

Like mothering, fathering begins in the womb. It is evidenced by the father's love and care of the mother and his genuine interest in the developing child. Although it is understood that the mother carries the responsibility for her own physical and mental health during pregnancy, there is no doubt that the attitude of the father has a significant bearing on the health of both mother and child. Neglect or abuse of the mother interferes with the harmonious interplay between the emotional, physical, and spiritual aspects of her person, thereby significantly reducing the nurturing she can give to her child within.

Psychiatrist Gerald Caplan, who has written extensively on mental health issues, states:

> We all know that a woman needs increased vitamins and proteins during pregnancy and that if she doesn't get them, she is likely to have all kinds of difficulties and complications. In just the same way, she needs increased supplies of love and affection and if she does not get them, she may have difficulty in giving love and affection to her child.[7]

In addition to providing a nurturing love of the mother that affects both mother and fetus, the father's choice of life-style has a direct biological influence on the child in utero. Scientists are now finding that it is not only the mother who can influence infertility, miscarriage, or genetic damage by her personal habits (e.g., smoking or the use of alcohol and drugs). Fathers should know there is real concern that sperm are vulnerable to unhealthy life-styles as well, and that damaged sperm can still fertilize an egg, with the possible result of birth defects for the child. Twenty to twenty-five percent of babies born with Down's Syndrome are a result of defective sperm. In addition, some toxins in the workplace may alter the chromosomes carried by the sperm thereby altering the genetic information conveyed to the developing embryo/fetus. The recent study by the University of Missouri offered the first convincing evidence that sperm quality varies significantly among regions of the United States. The quality of semen was significantly poorer in men from rural mid-Missouri than in males from urban areas and the authors of the study believe agricultural chemicals might explain the difference.

Because sperm develop over a three-month period "even if a man quits smoking, drinking, using drugs or if he removes himself from other toxins, most experts advise waiting three months before trying to conceive a child."[8] Preliminary studies also have revealed that cocaine attaches itself to sperm, and thus may carry the drug into the female reproductive tract. If conception does occur, the cocaine could affect fetal development.[9]

After birth, just the father's presence speaks unconsciously to the sexual identity of his children. His presence and companionship, and the emotional ties or bonding growing out of them, are an essential force that helps to determine whether his son or daughter assumes the necessary qualities of maleness or femaleness. Contrast these facts with the attitude of the father who described his child "as a stick of furniture until he can walk and talk."

Unless the father neglects his son's need of him, or other forces intervene, the boy will begin to imitate his father, both unconsciously and consciously. At first, it is in trivial things, but this pattern of imitation also extends to character traits, such as honesty and responsibility. In striving to emulate his father, he inevitably strives for masculinity itself. He becomes proud and eager to be a man.

Little girls, too, need their fathers. A father's love for his daughter should be the kind that pays tribute to her as a girl and affirms her femaleness. He can teach her the same things as he would a boy—carpentry or baseball—but always with a recognition and appreciation of her feminine strength. Fundamentally, of course, both sons and daughters need to feel that the father appreciates them as human beings with individual needs regardless of their sex, that entitle them to his consideration and respect. No matter how tomboyish a growing girl is in her play, or what career she chooses, she will develop her femininity as long as she learns to take pleasure in becoming a woman and develops contentment with her share in reproducing children, should she choose to do so. To develop in this way, a girl needs a father who is not merely attracted to women erotically, but who makes it clear that he appreciates a woman's distinctive femininity, who admits how he needs women, and who acknowledges the extent to which women enrich all living.

If a girl's normal development is to be assured, she needs a father to be a love object as satisfying to her as her mother, but in a complementary way. He can help her to be real and true in her everyday existence. He helps her to know and deal with the world as it is. If a girl's father disappoints her, or if he regards her as unattractive or unimportant, she unconsciously expects other men to disappoint her, too, and to reject her love. Distrust and competitiveness develop between her and the men who enter her life, in place of [the] mutual acceptance that is the only sound basis for marriage.[10]

For both boys and girls, the mother is the first human being to be loved. To both, she is perceived as the source of all that is good and nourishing. Sometime before the age of three, though with the realization that he is a boy, the male child is expected to convert to male identification. In order to do so the male child needs a warm, personal contact with his father, especially at this particular time, so that the transition is gradual. With such a fatherly influence, the boy is able to develop a private, individual sense of his own masculinity. However, when fathers are absent most of the time (whether at work or by choice) and when most of the child rearing tasks are left to mother, the son has little notion of what it is that males do. In such cases, at that particular point in time, the mother becomes the basis for the boy's sexual identity. This means that, in order to develop a male sexual identity, the boy must change direction and temper what he has already learned. In doing so, he must ignore his natural inclination, which is to follow the example of his mother and to model his behavior after hers. Indeed, some boys so thoroughly identify with their mothers that they will not or cannot switch to make identification. (Many more males fail in same-sex identification than females.) Some boys switch by consciously abandoning any feminine ways as a method to prove their masculinity. Some direct their resultant anger to the females in their lives, carrying this attitude throughout life. With growing anxiety about his maleness, the boy may repress his female-oriented responses and subscribe to the societally approved male myth of physical strength and aggressiveness.

Society's Influence

This societal male model is not an individual model of identification, but a cultural stereotype that is learned, not from contact with a male significant other, but from his mother, female teachers, primary school readers, male playmates, films, and television. As Kirkpatrick notes, for the boy:

> This is in contrast to his first sexual identification, [the mother] which was special and very individual. It is likely that, even after his reconditioning, many of his deepest, most 'natural' responses will be female…. But society is powerful. If a discrepancy arises between his natural inclinations and society's definition of maleness, he will likely suppress the former in favor of the latter; he will come to depend more on the cultural role and less on his spontaneous reflexes. The point is simply this: a sexual identity based on an intimate personal model (as it is for girls) is more secure than one based on a generalized abstraction (as it is for boys). In the second case…we do see many more attempts to compensate for a felt weakness in sexual identity by playing a sexual role to the hilt.[11]

Such compensation or gender defensiveness is often seen in present-day males. The more external the influence, the more rigid and defensive is the man.

Gilder defines the difference in male and female sexuality very bluntly:

> Women are tied to a long-range future oriented cycle of sexuality necessary for bearing and nurturing of children...[by contrast] the male pattern is episodic, present-oriented, in search of immediate gratification, unconcerned with long-term involvement, even frightened by them because they represent commitment.[12]

Unsure of their masculine identity, males tend to fear women and any relationship that may involve an unmasking of who they really are. Kirkpatrick also echoes this appraisal of masculine sexuality:

> Something in the heart of the American male...forever beckons him to the Marlboro Country and all it represents.... Males are always retreating to the woods or to women who won't tie them down.[13]

Despite the kernel of truth in these descriptions, such limited versions of masculinity and femininity have only brought confusion and dissatisfaction with society's version of sex roles. In the United States, child-rearing is still perceived as women's work.

A Jungian analyst, in comparing American males with English males, represented American child-rearing patterns for males as being tied to the mother rather than to the father. As a result, he felt that American males, on the whole, were insecure and dependent. Indeed, in many marriages, there is a need for constant attention by narcissistic males who are not secure in their masculine identity. Women in such a union have a difficult task to find time for their own development. Such dependent husbands often feel displaced when children are born and so fail to give their unconditional love to their offspring. Their struggle with jealousy limits the amount of undivided and pleasurable attention fathers can give to their child. Often, the wife is blamed and marital discord results, affecting the child even more. Most of these feelings are unconscious or denied so that emotional growth and resolution for all concerned is limited.

On the other hand, during pregnancy and the first six months of new life, husbands often feel ineffective and disposable but cannot articulate their needs. Some wives, absorbed in their new task of caring for a newborn, fail to notice the husband's dilemma. Misunderstanding occurs and family harmony is disturbed.

In American society it is the uncommitted male who is held up as a model, inevitable and innate. Men need to believe that their identity as males does not rely on episodic proofs of manhood but on an ongoing involvement in the formation and nurturance of family and society. They need to see themselves as important partners in parenting, the success of which is vital to society as a whole.

Sexuality And Violence

Society's sex role concepts are influenced by biology, parent-child relation-ships, and cultural reinforcement of traditional masculine and feminine role pre-scriptions. Presently, women are attempting to emulate the broadly drawn, short-term, focus-on-immediate-gratification masculine sex role just described, not only in terms of sexual behavior, but also in terms of violent behavior. Indeed, there has been an upward swing in the rate of female violence recently. Such behavior is at odds with women's sexual identity and is causing distress and con-fusion. By adhering to the value of the masculine mystique, we will pass along to the next generation a proclivity for violence.

Medzian, author of *Boys Will Be Boys*,[14] believes that the general tendency among boys for rough physical activity, self-assertiveness, and competition requires a form of social condoning and role model encouragement for it to become violent behavior. Boys as infants are often overstimulated. It follows then, that they become less sensitive in order to accommodate the handling they receive. In addition, boys with increased levels of testosterone become easily frus-trated and irritable.

However, I believe both sexes have a capacity for parental nurturance and abu-sive rejection of children. Generally speaking, to nurture or to abuse are choices based on the parents' own needs rather than on a fundamental difference in sex-ual identity. Studies show that our homes are the training ground for violence and its perpetuation. In a study comparing violent and nonviolent males, it was deter-mined that when parents taught their children to defend themselves, but also taught them that violence was not a way to solve conflicts, children learned by example to solve problems by reasoning. Conversely, when parents approve of aggressive behavior toward authority figures and peers, or when they model phys-ical abuse, they encourage aggressiveness in boys.

Children often model their code of conduct after their father even in the act of attending church services. He provides, especially through his work, a framework for the family—economic and social. He influences their sexual identity by the degree of nurturance he accords their mother.

Sex Roles And Masculine & Feminine Traits

Society says a boy is masculine and a girl feminine if they adopt traits that are the same as those of their same-sex parent. Traditionally, men are assumed to be dominant and aggressive, whereas women are pictured as passive, gentle, and nur-turing. Controversy continues whether men can nurture and women can be assertive. Such questions are divisive and lead nowhere. Traits such as these are possible in both sexes. Often, however, they have complementary expressions. It is quite possible, for instance, for a masculine son to be more similar to his mother than to his father in characteristics that the society does not sex-type, while retaining his masculine identity.

Consider, for example, the case of Mark, who was the son of a very athletic, extroverted father and an introverted, literary mother. Mark's father agonized over his son's lack of interest in athletics, telling him, "you'll never be a man." Mark had a high IQ, was interested in history, and preferred to be left alone to read, visit museums, and would later become an expert on the Civil War period. Mark had no difficulty in identifying as a male, and eventually had a successful marriage, once he had overcome the repercussions of his father's anxiety and disapproval. However, his self-confidence and ability to initiate were damaged. Had his father affirmed him as the unique individual he was, rather than judging him by the societal standard of maleness, Mark would have had a happier adolescence and as a result of more maturity—a more successful career.

The scientific theory of the way in which members of each sex develop masculine and feminine characteristics defies common sense and predicts that males are likely to grow up to be in many ways as much like their mothers as like their fathers. Both girls and boys are assumed initially to model after the mother, and boys must later shift their identification in order to become masculine. The time each parent spends with the child and the intimacy and intensity of the contact are pertinent to his patterning after one parent or the other.... We tend to become somewhat like people we are with a great deal even when we don't wish to do so, and that tendency is even stronger in childhood than in adulthood.[15]

Consider this scenario. The boy infant, if he experiences the love and presence of both mother and father from the beginning of his life, will unconsciously identify with the father whom he resembles. He will then have an opportunity to choose, without anxiety or sense of competitiveness, those traits from each of his parents that best complete and complement his genetic and biological makeup. As he forges his identity in the first few years of life, he will be fortunate to experience both masculine and feminine love, and will thereby internalize both. In this manner, the dual form of our sexuality, which has both male and female components, will be nurtured. Society fails to recognize this diversity in each individual and insists on sex-roles that promote divisiveness. Sex roles can even be in opposition to true sexual identity.

Transactional analysis, a theory initiated by Eric Berne, maintains that, as individuals, we all follow a life script. Another theory is that our unconscious records what it sees and hears. What is repeated becomes imprinted and often motivates our behavior. That is why I feel parental behavior is most important. A male child may consciously reject the behavior of the father but unconsciously record it and be motivated to act as his father did. This provides an inner conflict for the child. He will either act in accordance with his unconscious feelings or he will rebel, which will cause internal conflict. Confusion is the result of such inner conflict, and in extreme cases, such conflict can immobilize a person.

My work with a woman—we shall call her Joan—made the process of trait selection clearer to me. When I first met her, Joan was a 45-year-old woman who was unhappily married for the third time. She was the youngest of five children. She was unwanted at the time of conception, and was born into a busy household of growing children. Joan rejected her mother as a role model even as a child, becoming resentful of her authority and often being openly rebellious. To my mind, Joan sensed her early rejection, did not bond well enough with her parents to develop trust, and so was defensive and angry at an unconscious level.

As a growing young adult, Joan could not accept her mother as a role model, as the mother stayed at home and was, to Joan's way of thinking, submissive to her husband. Joan's image of herself included public recognition and wealth, as she was extremely talented. She admired her father's traits of vision and initiative as well as his ability to welcome challenges in life, and chose those traits as parts of her personality. However, anger at her father did not permit her to accept those traits freely until he died. That is when her sexual identity confusion became apparent. She had become sexually promiscuous as an adult and was suffering from alcoholism. Psychiatric treatment has helped her to come to terms with her unconscious choices to be like her father and her rejection of her mother. Currently, she is slowly building a good sense of self that was not adequately nurtured as a newborn. She now recognizes that failure to resolve these conflicts of trait selection and sexual identity contributed to hostile sexual relationships with her husbands. Her current marriage relationship is now being strengthened. Her sense of identity—as a woman with initiative and a competitive spirit—is being merged with a more reality-oriented sense of her femininity. She is no longer angry with her father. She understands her mother better, but her acceptance of her mother at the present time is less than wholehearted. Joan is still in the process of maturing, but is comparatively free of the confusion caused by faulty sexual identity development in her early years and her consequent lack of freedom to select parental traits that complemented her uniqueness.

Parental Harmony/Parental Strife

In further understanding trait selection by the individual child, we must return to what has been a recurring theme in this book—that the mother-father relationship greatly influences a child's development. A woman who is able to share the emotional and financial burdens of child-rearing with a supportive husband is more likely to be a loving, affirming mother than one who is constantly resentful of or angry at the child's father.

In congenial marriages, the mother communicates the father's viewpoint to the boy, buttresses the father's values and reinforces the father as a masculine model. The mother acts to conciliate the differences between father and daughter and can enhance a close relationship between the two. When a mother's ideal for her son is similar to her description of her husband, the boy models after the father and is highly regarded by his peers. The evidence suggests that when a mother is congenial with her husband she may subtly enhance her son's masculinity, and that when she is critical of her husband she may subtly encourage him to adopt more feminine characteristics. If the father is absent from home, the mother is in an especially strategic position to shape the child's image of his father. If the child was young at the time of a father separation, his impressions of his father are particularly vulnerable to manipulation by the mother. A mother's derogatory comments about the absent father can contribute to a child's developing a negative self-concept, and to his engaging in maladaptive behavior. In a boy, it can cause self-doubt; in a girl, distrust of all males.[16]

The societal myth of enmity between the sexes is strengthened and becomes part of the child's sexuality when s/he watches the parents frequently fighting and quarreling, or when one often speaks disparagingly of the other. In extreme cases, it leads to faulty parenting by both sons and daughters when they have their own families. Generational contamination!

Fathers As Authority Figures

The best evidence suggests that marriages that fail to meet the ideal of egalitarianism tend to be dominated by husbands, and that when husbands dominate, they do so more harshly than wives. Such marriages have an unfortunate influence of domestic violence in society.

From the father, children incorporate the prohibitions and values of society. To his child, he represents the authority of society for us all. Unfortunately, with some fathers, authority is synonymous with punishment. In reality, the word authority derives from the word author. The father, then, is the author or creator of life for the child. He brings a sense of the real world to each of his children and also inadvertently teaches them his means of coping with it. If he teaches force as a means to solve conflicts, the child will be open to violence; if he uses reason and love, the child will follow suit. A father's discipline will be effective if he follows the true meaning of the word it comes from—disciple (*L. discere*) to learn. Parents are the first teachers of children and children are eager to learn. They actually mirror what they see. We need to teach our children how to love and how to live. Punishment or a punitive attitude rarely accomplishes either of these goals.

Recent evidence on changes within the American family suggest, that compared to days past, fathers are less authoritarian and participate more in child-rearing and in household work previously designated as woman's work. Lynn reports that about half of adolescents reported father dominant households.[17] Father's authoritarian role in the family is lessening and the change seemingly comes through his own personality characteristics and the particular aspects of the marital union. Society has yet to support these changes.

In the sense that the father is the one who gives meaning to the world, he contributes to the spiritual development of his child. The father's attitudes give to the child a sense of God, how the world came to be, what all things mean. The small child's world is sharply limited or greatly expanded by what his or her father's habits and beliefs are. The child's sense of self, connection to others, and ability to contribute to the world in which he or she lives come from the father in a manner no other can duplicate.

That is why, for single parents, every effort must be made to find a substitute for fathers. Children need two parents or substitutes for both sexes. When there is only one adult in the home, there must be a stable substitute, if only to prevent the single parent from turning the child into a substitute for the absent parent.

Fathers As Providers

The father is generally regarded as society's representative within the family and the family's representative within society. Working and involved outside the home, he brings home his view of what is happening "out there." Unfortunately, many jobs have lost their meaning, and many men have come to spend long hours away from home in order to maintain their livelihood. Now, women are also breadwinners, sometimes earning more than their spouse and spending long hours involved with careers. Ironically, the family has become more important in giving life its meaning at a time when both men and women are forced to be away for long hours in order to support their families.

Having a job gives the male a chance to fulfill his societal masculine role as provider. If a man is jobless or very poor, he must seek other ways to validate his masculinity. A weak sexual identity leads him to make poor choices. In ghettos, men are denied the means to form or keep a long-term commitment to family or children, or even to society itself.

John Swanson says it well:

> With the advent of the industrial revolution, men began leaving home to go to work. A man's role came to be for the family rather than in the family…[Children] received the fruits of their father's labor but not much of their father. Some men often feel like work-horses harnessed with the burden of being family provider, trying to pull the family wagon up a muddy hill of financial debt. A wagon filled with an increasing load of mortgages, loan payments, medical bills, high-tech conveniences and maintenance and repair bills makes dreams of financial success seem impossible for all but the most wealthy. Today, two horses are often needed to pull the wagon, as shown by the increase in two-career families.[18]

Fathers As Empathy Enhancers

Medzian claims that: "Human beings, male and female, have significant potential for anarchy and altruism."[19] According to recent statistics, shortly after they reach the age of one, virtually all children begin to have some level of understanding of other people's experience and will attempt to help or comfort a person in distress. From age one and one-half to two years there is a great increase in altruistic behavior.

Researchers have found that, in older children, the degree of empathy and altruism is linked to maternal and paternal behavior. Nurturant involvement in child-rearing on the part of the father is linked to increased and enduring empathy in their children. Studies of mothers and children indicate that, when mothers are themselves empathic, they make their children emotionally aware of how hurtful behavior affects others. When mothers, nurtured and supported by the father, establish principled moral prohibitions, then children will be empathic and altruistic, as opposed to hurting others. A longitudinal study on empathy revealed that the level of paternal care was the single most important factor linked to the development of empathy.

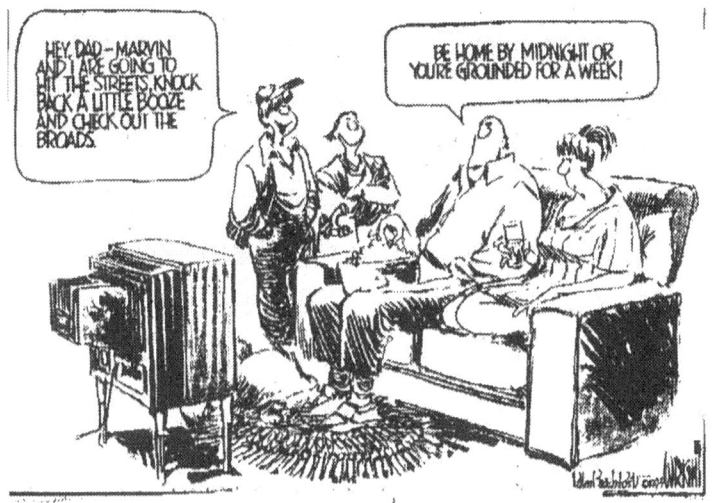

Figure 10-1 Cartoon—Marsh

Recent research on fathers and children has identified several emerging patterns:

1. When a father combines nurturance with dominance and a high level of participation in child-care, he increases the incidence of high masculinity in his son. A nurturant father also enhances his daughter's femininity in the long run. Research has revealed that this is particularly true of first grade girls and their fathers.

2. The way in which children develop masculine or feminine roles seems also to be related to the status of their father's work. Working men's children appear to sex-type earlier and have limited appropriate roles for both sexes. The father's role in the family is often formed by his work and his income. The more important his work is to society, the higher is the father's status. Higher income families also often have more liberal stereotypes of sex-roles. The children of these families have more opportunities to express their sexual identity in sports, music and the arts.

3. Major nurturant paternal involvement in child—rearing plays an important role in reducing male violence.

4. A father's influence is apparent in the vocational choices of both sons and daughters. Studies have correlated scholastic aptitude and style of thinking with the father's influence for both girls and boys. Interestingly enough,

mothers seem to be more influential in the creativity of their sons, whereas fathers have a greater influence on the creativity of their daughters.[20]

Conclusion

As a nation, we fail to teach men how to be good fathers, and we fail to use that ability as a measure of their masculinity. They are taught that fighting and competition are means to solve their problems. They are taught to confuse manhood and patriotism, because a sign of real masculinity is to support war. War gives an outlet to the male's inherent ability for strategy, to outwit the opponent, to be competitive. We fail to teach boys that to be a man is to use the strategy and competitive ability they possess to solve problems and create improvements in our communities. We fail to teach them that men have a responsibility to contribute to a peaceful and just society, and that this sense of responsibility must be passed on to their sons if society is to survive.

Our Creator, or nature (whatever entity the reader assigns the spirit), chose males and females to be formed in such a way that both were required to produce a new human being. It would follow, then, that both a man and a woman would be required to nurture this new human being until it is able to live on its own. Modern society has apparently relinquished both the right and responsibility for nurturing our young. Now, neither men nor women have time to nurture. Nurturing has instead been passed on to the phenomenon of daycare. Currently, plans are being considered to lower the standards of daycare. Minimum age for infant admissions changed from 6 weeks to 2 weeks; lower educational requirements for directors and license requirements for agencies changed from 2 years to 5 years. In upper New York State, county administrators are planning to reduce the amount a family can earn before being eligible for daycare. Who will the next generation have to hold on to?

Psychologist Ronald Levant told Newsweek: "Parents also delude themselves into thinking their daycare kids are doing fine simply because they "seem" to be. Children don't necessarily give outward signs of distress at early ages…. The effects of low parental interest show up later—on the shrink's couch or the police blotter."[21]

Approximately two years ago, a local columnist wrote a poignant story of his own need for a father that, to me, illustrates the importance of the bodily presence of a father. It underscores the concept that sons take in, consciously and unconsciously, the essence of the man they know as father.

Mike's parents separated when he was seven years old. As he expressed it, he had no input from his father on any of life's skills. "I had to figure it out for myself" was the way he put it. He went on to elaborate, "It's not just concepts like 'make sure you study something practical in college' or 'how to fix a car'. It is the way my father walks or reacts during a conversation, or approaches a problem— the patterns of his thought. I am now finding his ways of living from what I can learn of them."[22]

In brief…

❖ Men have a critical role in the formation of the sexual identity of both sons and daughters.

❖ Sex roles and sexual identity are not interchangeable concepts and can even be opposed

❖ Society develops stereotypical sex roles; it is men and women who develop sexual identity

❖ Fathers and mothers play an equal part in the development of a healthy identity of their child

❖ Men need to be taught a sense of masculinity that includes a responsibility to contribute to a peaceful and just society

❖ Violence is taught and perpetuated in the home.

Chapter 10—EndNotes

1 Medzian, Myriam, *Boys Will Be Boys*, Doubleday, New York, N.Y., 1991

2 de Chardin, Teilhard, *The Evolution of Chastity, Toward the Future*, (R.Hague, E. Traus), Harcourt, Brace, Jovanvich, New York, N.Y., 1975

3 Keen, Sam, *Fire in the Belly—On Being a Man*, Bantam Books, New York, N. Y., 1991

4 Ibid

5 Money, John, *Man, Woman, Boy, Girl*, John Hopkins University Press, Baltimore, Md., 1973

6 Kirkpatrick, Wm., Phd., *Identity and Intimacy*, Dell Publishing Co., New York, N.Y., 1964

7 Caplan, Gerard, *Principles of Preventive Psychiatry*, Basic Books, New York, N.Y., 1964

8 *Men Have Babies Too*, March of Dimes, Greater New York, 1992 Brochure

9 Reinesch, Dr. June, Column "Kinsey Report", *The Buffalo News*, November 1, l992

10 Wolf, Anna, W.M., *The Parents' Manual*, Simon & Schuster, Popular Library Edition, New York, N.Y., 1951

11 Kirkpatrick, op cit, p. 185

12 Gilder, George, *Sexual Suicide*, NY Quadrangle, NY Times Book Co, 1973

13 Kirkpatrick, op cit

14 Medzian, op cit

15 Lynn, David B., *The Father, His Role in Child Development*, Brook/Cole Publishing Co., Monterey, CA., 1974

16 Ibid, p.91

17 Ibid

18 Swanson, John, NCCMHC, "Sexism Strikes Men", *American Counselor*, Fall, l992, Vol 1, #4

19 Medzian, op cit

20 Lynn, op cit

21 Parker, Kathleen, Columnist, Orlando Sentinel, reported in *Niagara Falls Gazette* 5/17/99

22 Merrill, Mike, *The Buffalo News*, September 13, 1991

Section III

Pathway To Adult Sexuality

Chapter 11

Influence Of Infant Identity On The Formation Of Adult Sexuality

The attraction of man for woman and of woman for man can be profound, a thirst for tenderness which nourishes itself through sexuality and which leads to it. But, for that sexuality to be truly human, springing up from relationship and strengthening it, people must have a clear awareness of their identity, knowing who they are and what they wish to make of their lives…. Genital sexuality lived as covenant serves life; through it the family is built in the service of the little one, the child.[1]

Jean Vanier, Author

Sex may bring pleasure or joy, but not identity. In fact, we are able to lose ourselves in loving sexuality only to the degree we have found the self elsewhere. It takes a very secure person to surrender to another in love.[2]

Sam Keen, Author

Marie Jahoda, as a member of the fact-finding Committee of the White House Conference on Childhood and Youth, in March of 1950, defined a healthy personality as one who: "actively masters his environment, shows a certain unity of personality, and is able to perceive the world and himself correctly."

I like this definition because it expresses a certain balance of individual and environment, and implies a psychological integration within oneself and with the individual's place in the world. However, it falls short of expressing the fullness of the third dimension of a healthy personality—our spiritual dimension.

For a more personal and deeper explanation of a healthy personality, we may turn to Joan Borysenko's description:

> The psychospiritual work of a lifetime is twofold. First, we must become aware of our different personalities—those in the light as well as those in the shadow—so that we can walk through life as a whole person without waging...inner wars.... This is called psychological integration and wholeness. We have met our shadow, accepted our various parts, and learned to function as a coordinated being using all the different parts of our personality.
>
> Second, we need to recognize that even this well integrated personality that we call me—formed to serve our needs and acting as a vehicle through which we can experience life and express the potential within us—is still not who we really are. It is not the essential Self/Soul unit or center that is with us from birth and that...appears to accompany us after bodily death. When we experience ourselves as this essential center organized around the Self, rather than as any one of our roles, we can function optimally, unimpeded by fears and desires—[or] as the apostle Paul describes it, "in the world but not of it."
>
> Self realization has also been called enlightenment because it ends the illusion of faulty identification with our ego roles and awakens us to a more basic, enduring identity in which we feel safe, secure, loved and capable of radiating these qualities to other people.[3]

Added to these perceptions of a healthy personality is Kenneth Keniston's idea that an ethical sense is really an extension of one's sense of identity:

> When an ethical man violates his own ethic, he feels not guilt but a sense of human failure, a kind of existential shame that he has not been who he thought himself to be.... His ethical sense is a part (often the heart) of his central and best self.[4]

An ethical sense requires an ability to differentiate one's self from one's culture and to find a unique identity as an individual regardless of community mores.

To become an integrated adult then, we must have:

1. awareness of self
2. a lack of ongoing inner conflict
3. responsibility for our actions, both good and bad
4. a recognition of the Spirit (Light, soul, spiritual capacity) within us
5. an ability to act in an enlightened manner toward ourselves and others from a basis of love.

I believe that becoming such an integrated adult depends largely on the introduction to love afforded by our parents during the years zero to three, the years of greatest growth in all of life. Without unconditional parental love, the battle to wholeness is fraught with overwhelming odds.

The process of becoming whole is an enduring cyclical, generational movement. If our parents are loving, we become loving, and we then pass this love on to our children who, in turn, give a similar legacy to their children. As a result, our whole society benefits and becomes a community. Our world is cooperative and friendly—we become a peaceful people.

I am not speaking solely of affection or feeling when I speak of love. Love encompasses the recognition, as Borysenko reminds us, that the Spirit of Love is within us and is the basis of our ability to love.

In a talk given by author Robin Casarjean in Buffalo, New York in the fall of 1991, she defined love as

> …no more or no less than the natural expression of our own fullness of self-acceptance. Until we can accept all of who we are without judgment, together with the glory, we are not able to fully love.[5]

If we accept that we are both of value and imperfect and at the same time inseparable from Divine Love, we will love each other and our children. We have become mature adults.

Mothers and fathers, then, must come to a degree of maturity and self-acceptance before they can fully accept the responsibility of parenting. The beginning of such mature love is passed to the infant and in a nonverbal, vibratory manner to others. The greater the parent's ability to love, the greater the heritage of the child. It is the "thread of Divine Love"[6] that attracts and communicates. It is strengthened in the child in early love. If not thwarted, by faulty parental or other adult influences, this ability stays with the individual to adulthood.

The preceding chapters have attempted to explain the establishment of sexual identity in the first three years and its importance in building a sense of self, both psychologically and spiritually. In this chapter, we will attempt to outline the stages of growth in which sexual identity changes and matures. It is not the purpose of this book to outline the stages of sexuality. What is important for all of us to know is what a powerful effect loving parental care in the first three years has on later stages of adolescence and young adulthood.

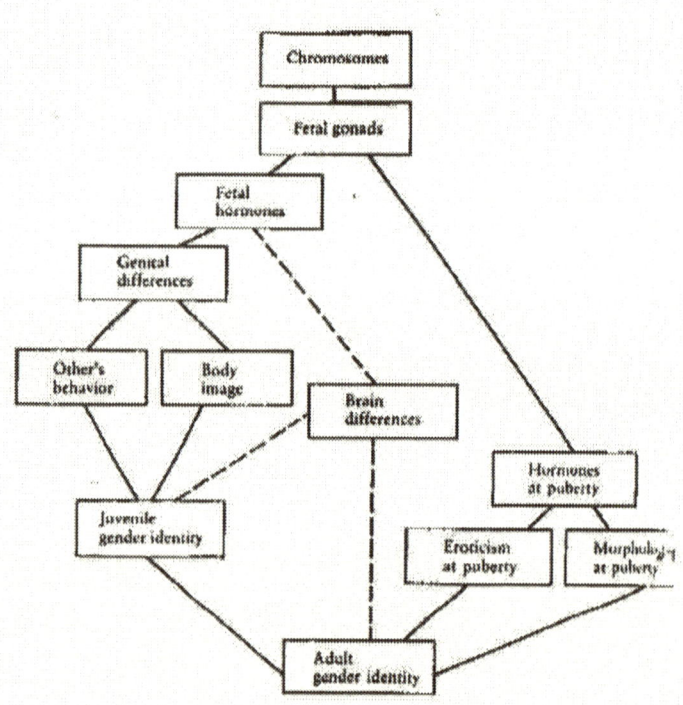

Figure 11-1 A graphic illustration of what we will attempt to briefly outline is found in Lewontin's biological blueprint of the pathways from conception to adult gender identity. From (Human Diversity, p.140 Richard Lewontin)

Infancy

Infancy is a time of normal dependency on an all-powerful provider whose presence and care ideally result in reassurance, pleasant taste sensations, inhaling, imbibing and digesting. Faith and trust are developed through the sensual and intimate components of the first mother-child relationship, which is the forerunner of adult sexual intimacy. The better the first relationship, the greater the capacity as an adult for intimacy with or without sensuality.

As we have already noted, a child's neural development, if influenced by negative or indifferent maternal attitudes, can result in aggressiveness and lowered mental capacity. This can occur when an infant is deprived of breastmilk and close body and skin contact with the mother.

Erikson notes that frustration in the early oral stage of infancy can engender feelings of being left empty, of being no good. It can create a cruel need to get and to take in ways that may be harmful to others. Such frustrations can give rise to addictions and destructive behavior in later life.

Integration, states Erikson, of all areas of the oral stage results in an adult who combines faith and realism.[7]

Toddlers And Preschoolers

In this modern economy, where time is money, it is easy to see the effect of tight schedules. When we have to hurry children to daycare or the sitters so as to be on time for the job, what do we do to the developing will of our children? They will perhaps be taught orderliness and punctuality, but their sense of choice and autonomy—the development of which is critical at this age—may be damaged. Infants may spend hours in car seats while the caretaker parent does errands or chauffeurs siblings.

At this critical time when our children are building a sense of autonomy, we as parents can easily instill in them a sense of shame and doubt by labeling natural maturation behavior as mischievous and willful. Consider the fact that this is a time when the muscle system is maturing. At this stage, children learn to coordinate such highly conflicting muscle patterns as holding on and letting go, both physically and psychologically. Still dependent, children learn to apply this concept of holding on and letting go to their developing sense of autonomy. Sometime they will be fearful and sometimes they will go out on their own. They have strong feelings inside which pull them about and which cannot be easily controlled. Their urges to *do* are new to them, and these urges lead toddlers to face new situations and experiences that may be frightening because they are not used to them. In the middle of exploration, they will frequently return to their parental "anchors(s)" as the person(s) from whom they derive the greatest sense of security and well-being. They seek the comforting familiarity of their parent(s) again and again, a security that daycare staff cannot supply to the child. Being able to say no to a familiar loving parent who understands the child's present stage of development, helps toddlers to separate from others and is one of the mechanisms that helps them become more and more aware of themselves as individuals.

As Erikson states, when the child has internalized the image of his mother "to an inner certainty as well as an outer predictability, he will be able to let go."[8] He will have taken one further step towards independence.

The aim of parents at this stage should be to develop in the child a sense of self-control without loss of self-worth; this, in turn, will result in a strong sense of autonomy and pride. By contrast, a loss of self-control, fueled by a sense of muscular impotence and parental overcontrol, brings a sense of doubt and shame that then has to be dealt with in adulthood.

If parents are firm and tolerant with their children, they in turn will be firm and tolerant with themselves. If children are encouraged to feel proud about their increasing autonomy, they will grant autonomy to others.

By age three, children have established a beginning sense of identity as either a male or female—a core gender identity. On an undifferentiated level, children then begin their first encounter with a desire for the opposite sex. Boys "fall in love" with their mommy, declaring their intentions to marry this most important person. Girls are equally determined to marry their daddy.

The child needs to establish a sense of identity as a boy or girl (an inner conviction that one is a boy or a girl) as a firm grounding for ongoing sexual development before this so-called Oedipal stage. This establishment of identity is the process we have been attempting to describe in preceding chapters. With continuing maturation of a strong sense of who they are; with models of mature parents who love each other and show their affection for one another, children see the reality of the situation and give up the goal to marry Mommy or Daddy—one more step toward identity.

The most difficult part of this passage for the child, I believe, is overcoming fear of the loss of the same-sex parent. If Jane loves her Daddy enough to want to marry him and believes she may be successful in doing so, she fears the loss of the love of her mother. If Bobby marries his mother, in his eyes, he loses the comradeship he has developed with his father. It is a time of considerable tension. It is easy to comprehend how this period often is unsuccessfully navigated by the child who is the offspring of an unhappy marriage or who lives with tense, or often absent, parents.

Constant sibling rivalry within the family is another cause of failure to establish early identity. The necessary sense of attachment or connection is strained, and anxiety develops as the child becomes unsure whether s/he is loved and whether, therefore, s/he is "OK". Moreover, in single-parent families, the absence of one parent—and the attendant lack of one gender model—poses a difficult problem for the child to overcome.

Hostility of a parent toward a child is still another obstacle. Such hostility thwarts any sense of goodness in a child while creating defensiveness and fear. There is a great need at this time for loving interaction between both parents with the child, and a mutual understanding of the child's unfolding sexual powers. With the need to be like the same-sex parent now becoming evident, children need to know that the physical indication of their sexuality will grow to be like those of Mommy or Daddy, with similar functions and behavior. This gives children a sense of direction for their lives. Johnny needs to know that he will grow big muscles like his Dad, that his genitalia will be similar, that he will likely have a family to care for and some kind of life's work. Ellen needs to know that she will have breasts to nourish her own babies and the organs to birth them. She also needs to know that she will have the same opportunities as her brother to learn and develop her abilities. It is reassuring to the child to know that there are differing sex roles that need not be stereotyped and to know how they, as an individual of a particular sex will develop. Each child has a singular capacity to receive this information. Each family has a pattern of communication that is distinct. Sex education is and must be a continuing and dynamic course of instruction in love, affection, and attention. Ideals are best taught as a day-by-day process "a dynamic growing set of values entwined with deep understanding that comes through example."[9] The important thing is that this knowledge be shared.

This knowledge of self as a boy or girl, as a person who has some control of self and environment, as lovable and loved is initiated between the years of zero and three.

Once this internal hurdle of the identity has been overcome, children are then ready to explore the outside world with new enthusiasm. They have determined, for the present at least, that they are OK, that they are either a boy or a girl, and that they live in a safe environment in which they can grow and choose friends. What marvelous progress this is when you consider that the child has also moved from physical helplessness to being able to walk, talk, think, laugh, and play, and that he or she is on the way to becoming a social being able to relate to others!

This sexual identity differentiation, with its growing capacity for trust and autonomy, is the agenda of the preschool child. If it is successfully completed, the child brings to school a full readiness for learning and a lively curiosity to explore a new world.

6 Years—Puberty

In normal development, the onset of puberty may occur as early as 9 years of age or as late as 14 years. The years before puberty have been labeled the latency period in sexual development. Such labeling often leads parents to believe that nothing is happening in the development of the child's sexuality. I prefer to view these years as a period of unfolding—of a deeper sense of gender identity; of a clearer sense of what masculinity or femininity means; of the child in affirmation of himself or herself as lovable; of his or her identity in terms of ego and gender.

During this stage, there is tremendous growth and development of the physical body, especially noticeable in terms of height and weight. Motor skills advance and are strengthened. The facial features lose their baby contours and are predictive of what the child will look like as an adult.

At the same time, unique personality characteristics take shape. The child's ability or lack of ability to make contact with others grows; special interests are chosen and skills are developed.

Both consciously and unconsciously, children at this age continue to select the traits displayed by their parents, especially the parent with whom they have the most contact.

The spiritual dimension of children grows as they seek meaning in what they see and experience. Why is the sky blue? What makes trees grow? Who made me? Where did I come from?

Leo Buscaglia captures the immensity of growth during this period:

> Children are total potential. Even when basic expression is mastered, children are still mainly a copy of the others in their lives. Yet already in the specialness of their receptivity and environment, their unique selves are being formed.[10]

Montessori also succinctly expresses the growth of these early stages in the following progression:[11]

I am what I am given.
I am what I will.
I am what I imagine I can be.
I am what I learn.

In the formality of school, some of the dreams and goals of children are often misinterpreted, or even lost. Part of the art of teaching is allowing the student to learn.

Unfortunately, conformity, rather than original thinking, is often the thrust of our present school system. Montessori warns educators to beware of indoctrination rather than developing the child's own uniqueness. She does not mean there should be no presentation of factual knowledge. Her warning emphasizes the development of the process of learning and thinking as critical.

Rachel Naomi Remen, medical doctor and psychotherapist, observes that spores found in mummies over a thousand years old that have unfolded into plants when given the opportunity of nurture. She uses this metaphor for children.

> When no one listens, children form spores. In an environment hos-
> tile to their uniqueness, when they are judged, criticized, and
> reshaped through approval into what is wanted rather than sup-
> ported and allowed to develop naturally into who they are, children
> wall the unloved parts of themselves away. People may become
> spores young and stay that way throughout most of their lives. But
> a spore is a survival strategy, not a way of life. Spores do not grow.
> They endure.[12]

An apt description of many of our children in our elementary schools today!

In addition, during these years children further develop their spiritual capacity as conscience, the basis of which we agree was formed in earlier years. They hear its small voice, feel guilt, and are fearful of punishment. The idea of God takes a more defined shape, often taking the same psychic form as that expressed by parents or religious. Care must be taken by both to avoid arousing guilt over physical sexual matters at a time when curiosity and experimentation are compelling motives. Discipline should be loving and firm, as the children learn the value of their parents from the boundaries they provide, from the limits that are set, and from what opportunities for learning they are offered.

As is now more widely recognized, discipline must teach a recognition of consequences, rather than using punishment as a method of control. Parents as the authors of life provide authority best through the teaching mode. And teaching a child to recognize consequences is an important part of sexual development.

For me, the most graphic illustration of what a child needs to be taught was expressed by Dr. Ray Helfer, pediatrician and author of *Childhood Comes First, A Childhood Crash Course for Adults*.[13] In speaking to a group of parents at a local high school, he described the course of development from child to adult as a trajectory to the moon. He used this analogy because the child's point of origin was known but the end of the journey and the environment at the time of adulthood years later was unknown. To make the journey, the child needed to be taught and to learn three things:

1. The difference between feelings and actions. The ability to sort out how one feels and then to decide how to act is a critical skill; that is, if one is angry or sad, one must first acknowledge those feelings and then decide what to do about them. Helfer tells the poignant story of his eleven-year-old son who loved to go bike riding with his best friend. One day, the

friend pushed Dr. Helfer's son off his bike. He fell and was shaken and bruised. When he reported the incident to his father, Dr. Helfer asked him how he felt about it. "Are you mad?" he queried. "No" replied the boy, "I am sad. You get angry when someone pushes you off your bike, but when your best friend does it, you are sad." "What do you intend to do about it?" pressed the father. "I haven't decided yet," was the boy's reply as he rode away to think it out. Clear thinking for an eleven-year-old!

2. Who is responsible for what? Defining areas of responsibility for the child helps to reduce, if not eliminate, many guilt feelings. Children often feel guilty because their parents fight, or they may feel responsible if some tragedy strikes. Getting a clear picture of that for which an individual is responsible is a characteristic that is most valuable in developing maturity.

3. Decision making. How to make a decision is a skill that even many college students lack. If we are to help children make choices, they must be taught the process early in life so that they can eventually make important life choices. Dr. Helfer suggests that choices should start early, perhaps with deciding what flavor of ice cream to have. Again, parents need to distinguish for the child which matters are the subject of choice and which are not. That means that the parents must have a clear understanding of their own priorities.

In the *Heart of Evil*, Eric Fromm says that small choices often start us on a road to unhealthy habits without our awareness of the implications.[14]

The characteristics critical to growth during this period continue to evolve. Companionship with the parent of the same sex or a teacher or neighbor is most important at this time. It helps the child identify with another in a spirit of equality of tasks, and equality of worth.

Initiative, enjoyment of competition, insistence on goals, and the pleasure of conquest are also part of the maturing process during these formative years. Boys usually approach such traits with a head-on attack; girls are often more interested in making themselves attractive. All of these are prerequisites for masculine and feminine selection of social goals and for the perseverance to attain them.

Childhood activities are the work that develops the adult. As a sense of industry is formed, with it comes the first stage of the division of labor for the sexes and equality of opportunity. At this stage, both parents and society plant seeds and place obstacles for their growing child, often unconsciously. The reality of life's circumstance alone can restrict opportunity for growth. The more limited the vision of the parents, the less equal opportunity for their children, especially girls.

Teen Years

Many people regard puberty—the beginning of adolescence—as the beginning of sexual development. The reader, I hope, will realize that the foundation for sexuality has already been formed by the time the child reaches puberty. As Erikson notes,

> …In puberty and adolescence all sameness and continuities relied on earlier are questioned again because of the rapidity of body growth which equals that of early childhood and because of the genital maturity that floods the body and imagination with all manner of drives.[15]

Just as during the critical growth period of zero to three years when the hormonal and related brain activity determined, to a large extent, the masculinity or femininity of the fetus/infant/child so, too, are adolescents' bodies subject to new infusions of testosterone and estrogen. Apart from the genitals, the appearance of prepubescent male and female bodies are virtually identical. Hormonal activity at puberty makes the adult sex differences more apparent. These changes are called secondary sex characteristics (i.e. pubic hair, breast development, change in voice). Internal changes are also profound. Girls begin their menses, and the eggs they produce are capable of being fertilized. Boys begin to ejaculate sperm that are capable of fertilizing eggs.

The neurohormonal influences on sexuality affect the teenager in many ways. For instance, the female hormones reduce the level of a certain chemical in the brain called monamine oxidase inhibitors. People with low levels of these substances are highly arousable. It is theorized that such brain changes explain why women are generally held to be more easily alarmed, stressed, or otherwise aroused than men. Women are particularly liable to emotional upset just before menstruation. Many grow depressed and irritable as the hormones hit the brain. Differences in brain function between the sexes help to explain why women generally tend to be more sensitive than men to taste, touch, and loud sounds, and why men react faster, yet are more readily distracted by novel experiences.[16]

Women have been known to score better on mental rotation tests when their estrogen levels are lowest. Similarly, men were found to perform better on such tests in the spring, when their testosterone levels were low, rather than in the fall, when they are higher.[17]

In addition to coping with body changes, the adolescent faces the task of attempting to consolidate their social roles. Adolescents bring to this task the sum of their experiences in childhood, usually only a fragmented knowledge of how their body works, and the sense of the world as either a welcoming or fearful place, depending on what they have learned so far. They are busy trying to integrate what they feel about themselves with what they appear to be in the eyes of others. They have to learn to connect what they have learned so far (mostly from their families) with the ideals held by the teenagers of the day. In their words, with what is "cool." They have to refight, on a different level, the crisis of the earlier years—am I lovable? am I masculine (or feminine)? who am I?

The identity (an inner sense of continuity) of adolescents can be either fostered and developed or diffused. Their sense of self worth is confirmed by a sense of "developing a defined personality within a social reality [they] understand."[18] Under ideal conditions, children have the nucleus of a separate identity that parents and their own uniqueness have fostered. Formation of core gender and ego identity that lasts through adolescence to young adulthood depends on the stability of the first stage of identity in infancy. Thus, if teenagers have experienced more deprivation than gratification in their early relationships, they will have an especially difficult adolescence. The impressions of the first stage are long forgotten by adolescence, but have an unconscious influence on development and behavior. When this early sexual and ethnic identity has not been formed, an adolescent youth tends to have only a confused identity. They reject the "cult" demanded by American adolescent standards. They act out and are labeled as delinquent—a label they accept, banding together with others so labeled, and adopting, as their identity, the identity of the group.

Another task of teenagers is to begin to separate from their parents. Again the influence of early bonding is felt. If children have not been nurtured sufficiently to develop a sense of self, they have little or no identity when separated from the parents. As a result, they may rely heavily on their peers. Giffen, in dealing with suicidal teenagers, describes their situation as follows:

> He will constantly search for the idealized parent figure. But his sense of self is entirely dependent on another, so when a youthful romance breaks up, he is left with nothing. "I feel like I lost a part of myself," he may complain. For the teenage romance may have been all that was left in his life. These relationships become as important to the young person's ability to live as milk is to an infant.[19]

This excessive dependency on friends often extends into the college years and beyond. One very pretty girl came to me to discuss her grief when her beloved grandmother died. After several sessions, we both agreed that her grief for her loss was genuine but could be borne. What was really troubling her was the fact that her friends had not supported her during this time and in fact, had seemed to ignore the incident. When we discussed how we are all have a fear of dying and have a tendency to avoid people who are dying, she began to understand that it was not that they liked her less, but that they were acting on needs of their own. With her sense of self somewhat restored, and a beginning identity strengthened, she was able to forgive them and take up friendship with them again.

So often parents misinterpret the signs of lack of identity and the extent of teenage depression. Researchers have found that one in five teens may suffer from depression. As Giffen describes it:

> Young people are not used to dealing with stress, and so they more easily convince themselves that no other person in the world has ever felt so awful. They are so afraid, so profoundly lonely in their suffering. They have not had enough experience with depression to know that, as dreadful as it feels, it will end; they will feel better. Too often, they see suicide as the only exit from their suffering.[20]

Giffen further reports that a study of a group of parochial school seventh and eighth grade students in suburban Philadelphia showed that almost one third of the students were significantly depressed and had thought of suicide!

In America, it is even more difficult to remain whole during this teenage period because one's upbringing is based on choice and the sense that, if given a chance, one can make it on one's own. With so many choices in the world of work, young people often find it difficult to settle on an occupation. They do not want busy work, but rather want to be engaged in something that is real—something that contributes to life around them. Our TV based culture assails this goal by preaching physical pleasure and leisure fantasies. Alan Moore, dean of the School of Theology in Claremont, California, clearly outlines the difficulties teenagers face:

> Young people today are socially pressured to be sexually active long before they have been prepared educationally and psychologically to cope with the deeply personal and highly charged nature of sexuality. The mass media are filled with romantic images of male-female relationships, and the myth prevails that "to be carried away" by one's sexual urges is a sure sign of love, which justifies sexual interaction…. A teenage boy faces the sexual pressure to "score" and in so doing, he reduces his partner to a sexual object. A teenage girl absorbs the idea that a woman is someone who is sexually desirable to a man, her worth lies in her value as a sexual commodity and her ability to control the male with the sexual favor she provides.[21]

In the throes of hormonal urges and body changes, with constant bombardment by concepts such as "safe sex" and "sex is success", teenagers often turn to sexual activity much earlier than their personality development can handle. The need for an early bonding with parents and continued support during the teen years is evident in Sorenson's work, *Adolescent Sexuality in Contemporary America*. Although parents cannot prevent the stress of adolescence, they can do much to help the youngster develop an equilibrium by understanding the forces that engulf adolescents' bodies at the same time that they are attempting to integrate present-day mores and trying to establish an independent self.

Sorenson terms the adolescent who seeks to find his identity in sexual activity as the *Sexual Adventurer*. In his nationwide search, 24 percent of boys and 6 percent of girls were so designated because they had an average of 16.3 sex partners. Sorenson attributed this behavior to the goals of enhancing self-image and contributing to the narcissistic makeup of any person who takes pride in sexual attractiveness.

Sexual adventuring provides the opportunity for what one might call "seed love": affection that one offers another in small but sufficient quantity from one's own self-love in order to generate as much possible reciprocation from one's partner in order to in turn feel that self-love.[22]

The findings of Sorenson's research echo the reasons that Giffen gives for suicidal impulse. They both bear out the importance of development of identity and self-worth in prior years, especially infancy. Because ego satisfaction and subjectivity are critical elements in the sexual adventurer's personality, he or she is usually far more preoccupied with self than with the sex partner.

> "[It] don't matter what he thinks about us, because there ain't no us…" The sexual adventurer does not want to be obligated to the sex partner in nonsexual aspects of their lives. The willingness to be obligated in other ways is usually a nonsexual function…. It is easy for the adventurer to feel love for another person when the parameters of a relationship are confined to sexual pleasure.[23]

Sorenson's research found differences between adventurers and other behaviorally labeled groups that corroborate the great need to establish a sense of self and self-love in infancy during the first stages of autonomy and trust. There were differences in self-confidence and self-esteem in teenagers who saw no connection between life's meaning and sex. The "adventurers" sometimes felt as though they were "addicted to sex, like drugs." Their relationships with parents and their identification with society were conflict-ridden, and sexual behavior was viewed as antisocial behavior. They felt that it was not normal to abstain from sex and considered the sheer physical pleasure of sex to be a means of lessening their feelings of being uptight. Their sense of personal responsibility seemed to be less than that of other behavioral groups, such as virgins and monogamists. As one such teen expressed it, "the way I am living right now, most of my abilities are going to waste."[24] He felt unable to change. In addition, group sex and drug abuse were more prevalent among the sexual adventurer group. Adventurers had a tendency to believe that what they were able to learn from sex they could apply to their personality in other aspects of living: "just as you learn to speak, you learn to feel."[25] This is an interesting observation since language development and core gender identity occur around the same time, usually the second year of life.

A recent Guttmacher study reveals that the number of teenage girls with four or more sex partners has doubled since 1971.[26] With the risk of AIDS and other sexually transmitted diseases, along with the danger of infecting infants, these statistics do not bode well for the future health of the nation.

Some teenagers experience a further tension—are they homosexual or heterosexual? With limited information, most people have been taught that heterosexuality is the norm and that we are all very similar. Parents can be helped in their understanding of this very controversial issue by learning that sexuality exists in all of us in varying degrees along a continuum, as was made clear by Masters and Johnson's continuity rating scale (Figure 11-2).

Kinsey Scale of Sexual Orientation

Heterosexual			Bisexual		Homosexual	
(100%)	1	2	3	4	5	(100%)
	A Few homosexual fantasies or experiences	More heterosexual fantasies or experiences than homosexual		More homosexual fantasies or experiences than heterosexual	A Few heterosexual fantasies or experiences	

Figure 11-2 From A.C. Kinsey et al, Sexual Behavior in the Human Female[27]

In addition, Bell,[28] (who studied 1500 individuals) suggests:

> …sexual preference is likely to be established quite early in life and that childhood and adolescent sexual expressions by and large reflect rather than determine a person's underlying sexual preference…. A child's display of gender nonconformity greatly increases the likelihood of that child's becoming homosexual regardless of his or her family background and regardless of how much the child identifies with either parent.

However, Bell also found that:

> for both men and women, poor relationships with fathers seemed more important than whatever relationships they may have had with their mothers. Homosexuals' generally negative relationships with their fathers and lesbians' [perceptions] of their fathers as detached, hostile, rejecting and frightening, displayed a very modest but direct connection to that gender-role nonconformity and to sexual elements of their development as well.... The exact nature of this paternal connection remains ambiguous—[it is yet unknown] whether a poor paternal relationship predisposes a son or daughter toward homosexuality or whether sons and daughters who are sexually different find it especially difficult to maintain good relations with their fathers.

Bell further stresses the need for more research on biological causes of homosexuality and on the "ways biological predispositions interact with social and environmental forces, in order to provide a fuller picture of how we come to be the homosexual or heterosexual people that we are."

Present research indicates that there are biological, psychological, and spiritual reasons for sexual variation. The influence of each varies with each individual; thus, stereotypes are confusing and shortchange the uniqueness of the individual. Occasional homosexual activity is a means of sexual exploration in many developing youngsters. Some adolescents, having experimented with homosexual activity, stay in that mode, feeling safer with a person of the same sex. Some use it as a method of relieving tension without reproductive complications.

A principal issue raised by homosexuality in both males and females has to do with what it means to be a man or woman. It goes far beyond the matter of feminism and equal rights and addresses itself to the basic issue of gender identity itself. Society must ask itself if its survival depends on a rigid conformity to gender roles and characteristics. Parents must question a set of values that too often include an insistence that their children be just like themselves.[29]

Sex education in school is no substitute for parental instruction. Sex education begins in infancy and the best way to teach a child is for the mother and father to love one another and to openly show affection. Day by day, positive attitudes about sex on the part of the parents present to their child(ren), a healthy picture of male and female interaction and gender differences.

With the life-building tasks of adolescence, it is no wonder that this time of life has been given such a dismal reputation. However, recent research, reported in the Journal of the American Academy of Child and Adolescent Psychiatry, argues that the widespread cultural dread of adolescence is largely undeserved. Studies show that many adolescents have positive attitudes toward their parents and are capable of abstract thinking. Studies also show that girls, in particular, and poor, minority and city-dwelling young people have much more difficulty in coping with adolescence. Vulnerability to peer pressure and a degree of self-centeredness, which are normal, become life-threatening when mixed with the guns, drugs, and disease that are often a part of today's culture. Parents are often misled that teenagers will grow out of their problems, but experience has shown that troubled teenagers need parental guidance and/or professional help. A 1995 school health survey of 2700 students recently found 58% of a local high school senior class was sexually active and 85.8% admitted to use of illegal substances. What does this portend for future generations?

In following the crowd, adolescents very often become isolated and fail to reveal their true feelings to anyone. This is a period when one should be developing attachments to both sexes so that one can proceed with self-definition and discovery of others. In doing so, one becomes aware of one's inner identity. Confidence and self worth increase. Often, adolescents fail to complete this state of identity before marriage. Very often, sexual intimacy is mistaken for real intimacy and the youngster, unsure of his identity, grows wary of interpersonal intimacy, instead of developing toward it.

Adolescence is the last and concluding stage of childhood. It is only completed when the individual has subordinated his childhood identification to a new kind of identification achieved by making friends and competing with his peers.

Young Adult Years

Young adulthood is the third critical period in the stabilization of a person's unique development, when separation from parents takes place. To review, the first separation known as individuation, as I have attempted to show, occurs by the time the child is three years of age; the second occurs during adolescence. Young adult separation occurs on a deeper level and is probably final. This does not mean that the child-parent relationship ends—it merely changes from one of dependence to one of interdependence. As one person phrased it, "We are parents for life."

In the transition to adulthood, adolescents must become established as separate, integrated individuals with the capacity to form meaningful relationships; they must develop the ability to be alone and to function autonomously. The balance of autonomy and relatedness is extremely important and is a theme that will recur frequently in any discussion of various relationships. In order to understand this process, one must turn to the individual's early development and trace the implications of earlier phases for adulthood. Blos has written that the chief developmental task of adolescence is the "second individuation process." He compares it to the first individuation phase, described by Mahler as occurring around ages one to two, at which time:

> ...one attains a sense of self and a sense of constancy of those around one.... The most important relationship to a developing human being is the mother-infant relationship. Individuation, in the sense of psychological separateness, can only occur if a prior relationship with one who loves unconditionally has already been established. The issues of individuation and autonomy are reworked during adolescence and early adulthood and possibly during the entire life cycle. (see Figure 11-3) A further aspect of the establishment of autonomy is the process in which the individual's own psychological boundaries become more clearly established and strengthened. This in turn enhances the capacity to form close, intimate relationships since the threat of losing oneself in a relationship is lessened. The ability to relate as a separate person with a firm sense of self is only gradually achieved and adolescent relationships themselves form the crucial context in which it occurs. The ties to the family are not ruptured but are redefined.[30]

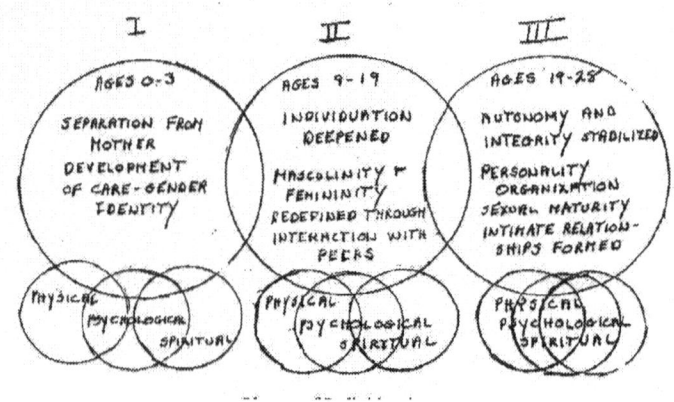

Figure 11-3 Phases of Individuation (Vaughan)

In the final phase of individuation, the development of cognitive skills is important. The authors of *Friends and Lovers* outlines the parallel development of cognitive skills and relationship progression in young adulthood (Table 11-A). At first glance, these components seem to have little in common, but they are actually closely linked.[31]

	Cognitive Development	Relationship Progression
1	Absolute approach, there is one big truth	Total Acceptance or rejection of parents, teachers, and authority figures
2	Disillusioned, all views are relative,	In-group members are OK; one as good as the other Gradual experience with "out" group, forms tentative friendships
3	Develops ability to evaluate theories; choose own values, set priorities and develop capacity	Evolve stronger relationships with fewer people; begins commitment

Table 11-A Cognitive and Relationship Progression (from Friends and Lovers)

From this research a picture emerges that a high level of emotional responsiveness may be associated with advanced cognitive organization.

All of the cognitive skills that were found to be related to the ability to respond with more emotion are marks of a highly organized awareness—an awareness that might be governed by a well-structured system of values, thoughts, and beliefs, but not by momentary excitements.[32]

This finding is gaining more acceptance with new discoveries of how our brains are influenced by our physical state of health and the state of our own emotions. Unfortunately, colleges pay much more attention to the cognitive development and very little to relational development, leaving students on their own with little or no information to guide them.

In the young adult...after considerable vicissitudes, the shifting ego-ideal and sense of self will ideally stabilize. Under these circumstances, self-esteem will become more firmly established, although fluctuations in self-esteem continue throughout life, rising and falling in relation to external success and failure, or sometimes independent of objective events but in reaction to the lifelong internal process of measuring one's self against one's ego-ideal. The internal process is never the only determinant. People always remain somewhat responsive to other's regard of them, but in adolescence, outside opinions are especially powerful. As the transition to adulthood is achieved, most individuals become less vulnerable to the opinions of others, in part because their sense of self has consolidated.

At the same time, as these social influences are at work, the individual sense of gender identity, formed in early life, is developing, further resulting in adult sexual choices. All the influences of early nurturing, acceptance, trust, autonomy, submission and receptivity are a part of adult sexuality, including orgasm. All of one's life is a reworking and expression of elements of identity in sexuality.[33]

In counseling young adults and in encouraging them to sort out relationships and to establish their own identity more clearly, I used a device created by Dr. Helfer and presented in his book, Childhood Comes First (Figure 11-4). In this construct, the length of each segment relates to the number of relationships in a particular category that one might have in a lifetime.

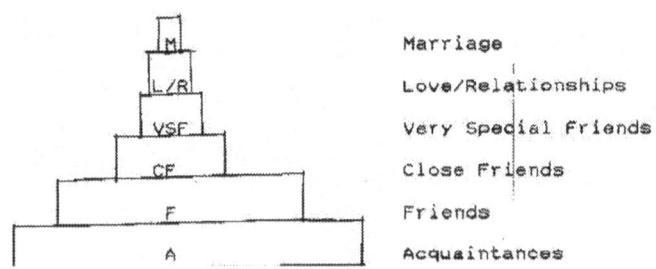

Figure 11-4 Relationships (Helfer)

In considering each level of friendship and intimacy, these young adults were asked to assess the importance of each type of relationship and to decide in which type sexual activity could or should occur. This exercise helped them sort out their values so that their whole sexuality could be involved in a relationship, not merely their physical sexual response. It also served to point out that the last two segments are not necessary in order to function well as a healthy adult—that it is possible, to live alone or with a close friend without moving into a sexual relationship.

Adult Relationships

Just as in infancy, the physical, psychological, and spiritual aspects of a person play an interlocking part in adult relationships. To attain intimacy in a relationship, whether erotically sexual or not, one must have a solid sense of self. One must be able to trust that the self will not be destroyed in allowing dependency on another at a particular time, or when relinquishing control. It is equally important that the other person be seen realistically. One must not be distracted by neurotic misconceptions of the other that can lead to defensive interaction. In a sense, this means that the other's needs must be maturely assessed and granted the same importance as one's own.

Similarly, as stated in *Friends and Lovers*, the experience of intimacy reflects a struggle characteristic of adolescence, that is, between the wish to keep old attachments unchanged, i.e. for old ties to remain, and at the same time the wish for change, for separateness and for developing one's own identity, all of which are enhanced by relationships with new people.[34]

Differences in a mature intimate relationship can be acknowledged, but often are temporarily ignored in seeking the goal of being able to love or to be loved as one was as an infant. Again, the identity factors of early infancy—lovability, gender identity and autonomy—are all involved in the development of intimacy. Indeed, the dance of mother and baby described in a preceding chapter is a forerunner of the dance of sexual union.

If the relationship is built on genital sexual feelings alone, the same factors are involved except that, instead of commitment to the relationship, the goal is specific drive release and satisfaction. Modern society has glorified this type of intimacy with the presumption that if one is not sexually active, one is unhealthy or not a whole human being.

The need for commitment as an integral part of an adult sexual relationship is beautifully expressed by Sam Keen, who refutes this modern dictum:

> Sexuality is wonderful and terrible because it is our link with the creative power of Being itself…. If we ever lose sense of the ontological fact that human sexuality is defined by a situation that implicitly involves the triad of man-woman-child, we neglect something of the spiritual dimension of sexuality.[35]

In maturity, our developed spiritual capacity allows us to believe and to trust in someone higher than one's self and is the forerunner of the ability to transcend oneself either in love of others or love of God.

One of my alcoholic clients confessed to me that he used the bottle in place of prayer. He was aware that he did this, but his anger was so strong that he found it difficult to do otherwise. He was isolated from his father, heartsick about it, and was unable to bring about reconciliation. He needed the help of a power greater than himself to overcome his anger but he couldn't pray and sought the bottle to overcome his pain.

Everyone feels the call to integrity of person—which includes our capacity to acknowledge a power greater than ourselves. We all have a vocation to become all we can be. We have a commitment to be a whole being. If we shortchange ourselves by wrong choices, or if our choices are tainted for us by lack of (or not enough) unconditional love, we are forever seeking the peace of integrity, often trying to find it in alcohol, promiscuity, and abuse of others, especially children. Spiritual development plays an important part in commitment to our wholeness. Lack of spiritual development has resulted in the vacuum of meaning that haunts our time. Our spiritual dimension is increased by human love. In love, we learn to respect what we cannot understand. In love we learn there is mystery, the limits of which we cannot probe, whether the love is human or Divine.

Adulthood is attained when one is able to love—not only sexually—but "for the good of the beloved." Erikson calls this generativity or "the interest in establishing and guiding the next generation."

Although Erikson is quick to add: "there are people who...because of special and genuine gifts absorb their parental responsibility in other forms of altruistic concern and creativity." In addition to generativity, adulthood, according to Erikson, also requires the ability to work and to develop a creative gift or skill but not to the extent that the person loses his ability to be a sexual, loving human being.[36] (see figure 11-5)

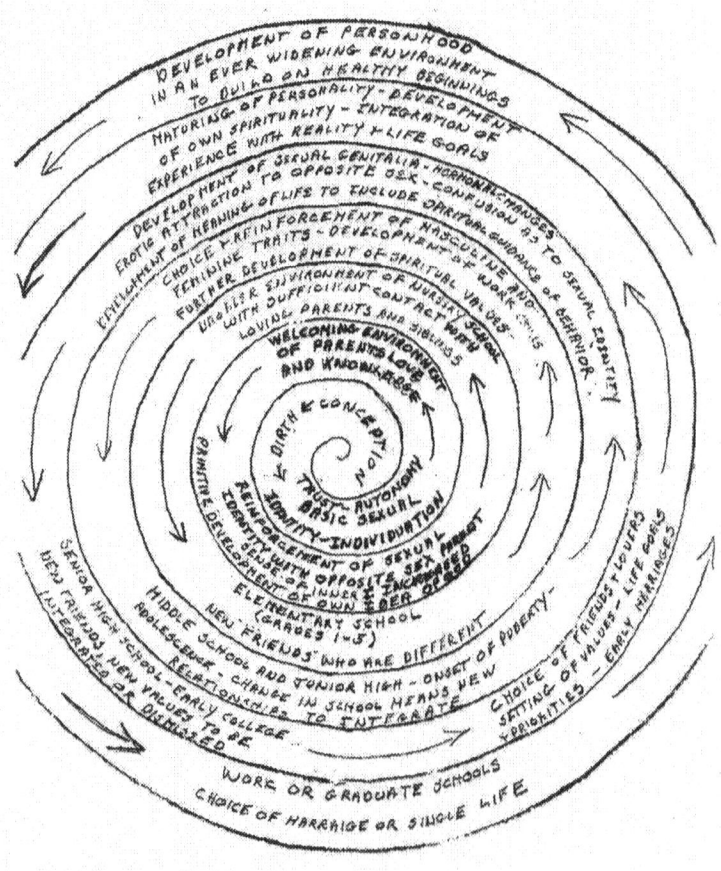

Figure 11-5 Spiral Growth (Vaughan) Adaptation of Bruner Theory

The second aspect of adulthood (the ability to work) has, in the past, been denied to many women. In an effort to correct this wrong, many women have come to dismiss the creativity involved in parenting and in making a home, and have instead sought fulfillment only in the same career avenues as men.

To explain what could be happening to the cultural feminine psyche, one must look to a hypothesis best expressed by Jung, a Swiss psychiatrist and a colleague of Sigmund Freud. Recall Money's view that, in gender identity differentiation of the brain after birth, neither the male nor the female system is totally and completely obliterated, but one merely becomes dominant over the other. For me, this underscores Jung's anima/animus theory that holds that all males have a feminine aspect to their personality and all females have a masculine component. In order to be a whole individual, these aspects have to be admitted to consciousness and developed. It is a difficult theory to understand and this book is not the forum to even outline it. However, a successful union of these diverse elements of personality increases the individual's creativity and ability to experience successful relationships with the opposite sex. Failure to do so restricts emotional development and leads to false projections being made on one's sexual partner (Figure 11-6).

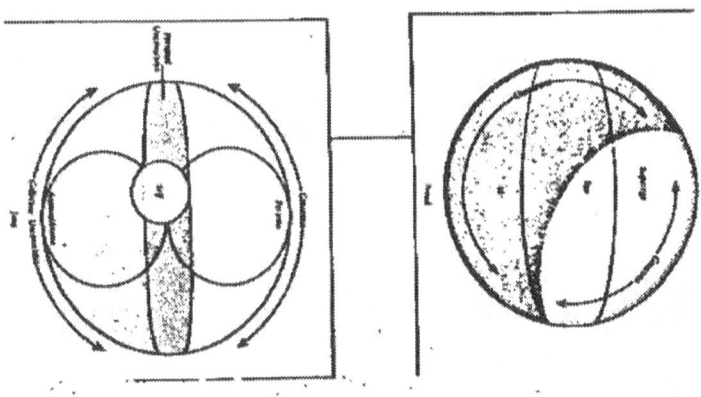

Figure 11-6 McGuire, Care and Feeding of the Brain, p.45.

Carl Jung was a disciple of Freud's, but broke from him on several key points. Like Freud, he retained the notion of a conscious mind and an unconscious mind for simplicity's sake, but he split the unconscious mind into two categories (1) an ever-shifting "personal unconscious," consisting of details and issues in our own lives that we're not consciously attending, and (2) a stable "collective unconscious," consisting of patterns, images, and issues that

are common to all humans and that shape how we reason, imagine, and live.

> The personality that emerges from Jung's conscious/unconscious mind has three major dimensions; (1) a persona, which is the face that the individual presents to the outside world; (2) a self, which is the individual's "true" identity; and (3) an anima (for a male) or an animus (for a female), which is the individual's "soul-self," a force embedded in the unconscious mind with which the individual craves union. The anima/animus is conceived as a sexual opposite (female for a male, male for a female) because of the yearning element involved in this soul-seeking and according to Jung, it plays a strong role in the individual's creative urge and search for a life-mate.

In returning to school at age 48, I was forced to reexamine my own adult beliefs. I found that I was very much a combination of my father and mother. I had copied similar traits from each but found that I had not properly integrated them into my own personhood. It was an astonishing revelation.

It is my belief that today's woman is looking to develop the masculine component of her personality at the expense of her feminine nature. She is becoming more extroverted, less inner directed, less receptive, less able to bridge the inner and outer world. With the sexes no longer complementary to one another, it leaves a gap in the attainment of wholeness for both men and women. It leaves no place at all for the child. Peace and integrity (wholeness) for the individual is no longer possible, especially for succeeding generations. Conflict and anxiety are projected, and the world becomes a maelstrom—our present state of affairs.

Both male and female adulthood encompasses a realization of one's own mortality; it also allows an adult a fresh look at one's parents, with loving acceptance that they were the ones needed in order to create one's uniqueness. It means an acceptance of responsibility for one's own health, life-style, and beliefs. Accepting of other life-styles, people with integrity have a firm sense of the dignity of their own life-style. They can be followers or leaders but they must be participants.[37]

Women are extremely important to the peace of the world, not only at the negotiating table or at the United Nations but in the ongoing development of their own creativity and integrity. Only then can they make a free choice to nurture their children—the fruit of a freely chosen union. Men must recognize the collegiality of such a union and cooperate in the realization of opportunities for all: fathers, mothers and children.

Lynn sums up our dilemma succinctly:

With marital roles undefined, with woman's knowledge of their inferior position made increasingly conscious by the dissemination of the Women's Liberation point of view, with men threatened by women's anger and by changing sex roles, and with both husband and wife adhering to the self-fulfillment ethic, the inevitable conclusion is that unhappy and broken marriages will increase. (Gilder, 1973; Levine, 1972). The marital heroes of our age will be those who have the integrity to define their own roles without the support of society, and who have the maturity and good will to maintain stable and loving marriages and give their children the love, security, and continuity they need. They will maintain perspective and will not become casualties…. [However] most people are not heroes…they lose perspective and stability as they are swept up by movements as their traditional cultural roots dissolve. As a consequence, the proportion of children who suffer the effects of conflict-laden homes will increase.[38]

It seems we have completed a circle. Remember, we began with the importance of relationships and how they extended from a beginning cell to the formation of community. It behooves us all to strive to be heroes—the alternative is unacceptable.

In brief...

❖ Growth is a spiral process, proceeding gradually from conception to maturity in an ever-broadening sphere, always building on prior growth and development.

❖ The growth of sexual identity formed in the early years as a result of interaction with parents, is later shaped and developed by interaction with peers and societal mores.

❖ The stronger the core gender identity and sense of self-worth the individual possesses, the more likely life will be true to the individual's unique needs and directed by creativity rather than social conformity or peer pressure.

❖ The personality traits one brings to the adult sexual union determines its success; physical compatibility is only one aspect.

❖ Education at home or in school should be directed to helping children understand and to cooperate with their own development in the three areas of physical, psychological, and spiritual growth as they mature.

❖ Satisfactory sexual relationships depend on the mature growth of all three dimensions of our personalities.

Chapter 11—Endnotes

1 Vanier, Jean, *Male and Female, He Created Them*, Paulist Press, Mahwah, New York, N. Y., l984, 85 and l989

2 Keen, Sam, *Fire in the Belly—On Being a Man*, Bantam Books, New York, N. Y., 1991

3 Borysenko, Joan, *Guilt is the Teacher, Love is the Lesson*, Warner Books, New York, N.Y., 1990

4 Keniston, Kenneth, "Moral and Ethics", *The American Scholar*, l965, vol. 34, p.628

5 Casarjean, Robin, *Talk on Forgiveness*, given at Hospice Conference, Hilton Hotel, Buffalo, N. Y., Fall, 1990

6 deCastillejo, Irene Claremont, M.D., *Knowing Women*, Harper Colophon Books, Harper & Row, New York, NY, 1974

7 Erikson, Erik, *Identity and the Life Cycle*, W.W. Norton & Co., New York, N.Y., 1959, 1980

8 Erikson, op cit

9 Erikson, op cit

10 Buscaglia, Leo T., *Personhood*, Chas. Block, Inc., Tharafare, N. Y., l978

11 Montessori, Maria, *The Child in the Family*, Translated by Nancy Rockmore Cirillo, Henry Regnery Co., Chicago, Ill., 1970

12 Remen, Naomi Rachel, *Kitchen Table Wisdom, Stories That Heal.* Riverhead Books, New York, 1996

13 Helfer, Roy, M.D., *Childhood Comes First, A Childhood Crash Course for Adults*, Self-published, East Lansing, Mich. 48823, l978

14 Fromm, Eric, *Heart of Man, Its Genius for Good and Evil*, Harper & Row, New York, N.Y., 1964

15 Erikson, op cit, pp. 94, 98

16 The Diagram Group, *The Brain, A User's Manual*, Berkeley Publishing Co., New York, N.Y. 1984

17 Sorenson, Robert C., *Adolescent Sexuality in Contemporary America*, World Publishing Co., New York, NY, 1973

18 Darrach, Forest Jacqueline, co-author Alan Guttmacher, Institute Study of Reproductive Health, reported in *Buffalo News*, 12/11/92

[19] Giffen, Mary, M.D., with Carol Felsenthal, *A Cry for Help*, Doubleday & Co., Garden City, New York, 1983

[20] Ibid

[21] Moore, Allen J. *The Young Adult Generation: A Perspective on the Future.* New York: Abingdon Press. 1969. Multicultural Resource and Research Center. School of Theology, Claremont, California

[22] Sorenson, op cit

[23] Sorenson, op cit, p.251

[24] Sorenson, op cit, p.252

[25] Sorenson, op cit, p.261

[26] Darrach, op cit

[27] Kinsey, A.C., et al, *Sexual Behavior in the Human Female*, Indiana University Press, Bloomington, IN, l953, 1998.

[28] Bell, Alan, P., Weinberg and W.K. Hammersmith, *Sexual Preference: It's Development in Men and Women*, Indiana University Press, Bloomington, Ind., l981

[29] Bell, op cit

[30] Silber, Sherman J. *The Male from Infancy to Old Age*, Charles Scribner Inc., New York, NY 1981

[31] *Friends & Lovers in the College Years*, formulated by the Committee on the College Student Group for the Advancement of Psychiatry, Published by Mental Health Material Center, New York, NY, 1983

[32] Sommers, S., "Emotionally reconsidered, The role of cognition in emotional responsiveness", *Journal of Personality and Social Psychology*, vol 41, p.560, 1981

[33] Friends and Lovers, op cit

[34] Friends and Lovers, op cit

[35] Keen, op cit

[36] Erikson, op cit

[37] Borysenko, op cit

[38] Lynn, David, *The Father, His Role in Child Development*, Brooks/Cole Publishing Co., Monterey, Calif. L974

Section IV

Can We Change?

Chapter 12

Creating A Society Viable For Children

On the other hand, students of history continue
to ignore the simple facts that all individuals
are borne by mothers; that everybody was
once a child; that people and peoples begin
in their nurseries; and that society consists of
individuals in the process of developing
from children into parents.

Erik H. Erikson,[1]

Americans have come to believe they are entitled
to all sorts of self-realization, gratification and
fulfillment—without strings, pain or
responsibility.... Meanwhile, it is the genuine victims
of misfortune, discrimination and injustice whose
experience is trivialized and ultimately drowned out...
Clinging to a sense of personal grievance is a poor
route to enhanced self-esteem.... A moratorium on blame
does not mean suspending the search for justice, nor
does it deny the complexity of society's problems.

Charles J. Sykes, Author[2]

Dr. Norris Hansell, a Canadian psychiatrist, places the essentials for life at seven. Each citizen needs, according to Dr. Hansell:

1. Food, oxygen and information of essential variety
2. A clear sense of self-identity, held with conviction
3. Persons, at least one, in persisting, inter-dependent contact, occasionally approximating intimacy
4. Groups, at least one, comprised of individuals who regard this person as a member
5. Roles, at least one, which offer a context for achieving dignity, and self-esteem, through performance
6. Money, or purchasing power, to participate in an exchange of goods and services in a society specialized for such exchanges
7. A comprehensive system of meaning, a satisfying set of notions which clarify experience and define ambiguous events[3]

Our founding fathers wished for us life, liberty and the pursuit of happiness. How does our society measure up in fulfilling these goals? Do we as individuals have these seven crucial essentials?

This chapter will speak to how these essential needs might be provided in our society, if we really care about our children.

First—The Setting: Where Are We Now?

Over the past twenty-five years, there has been a definite decline in the amount of time and attention parents give to their children. Sylvia Ann Hewlitt, an economist, figures the amount of contact time between parents and children has dropped by a "staggering 40 percent.... Today the average worker puts in six hours more per week than in 1973".[4]

Moreover, the world's anger, hatred, and destruction are growing at a far greater rate than its efforts for peace, love, and real creativity. Is it because we are ignoring the advice of Plato who declared: The right education must tune the strings of the body and mind to perfect spiritual harmony?

Let's take a look!

Dr. Joseph Beasley, in his book, *Betrayal of Health*, presents a very pessimistic view:

> For a significant number of Americans drug use must seem like a reasonable response to dead-end lives (For each person the reason

for such an attitude may be different). Young men and women who have developed in a malnourished, toxic womb, grown up on a poisonous environment on inadequate diet and received marginal or worse education have little to hope for in today's society. It is this pervasive malnutrition, toxicity and social disenfranchisement that fuels the drug epidemic…. In failing to recognize this most basic underpinning of the addiction epidemic, the war on drugs is missing the chance to have a real impact on the crisis and is indirectly fueling two of America's other serious behavioral problems—unsafe sexual practices and violence.[5]

In our violent society, the latest report from the Child Abuse Center indicated the number of abuse cases rose to over 3 million in 1994 up from 2.7 million in 1991, and 2.5 million in 1990. In 1991, 1383 children died from abuse or neglect, a 54 percent increase in six years. Of these deaths, 79 percent were among children younger than five years of age, and 54 percent were among those age one or younger. The mortality homicide rate overall for children under one year from 1950 to 1980 rose 69 percent.[6]

School-aged children fare no better. The American school, documented by the United States Senate Committee as long ago as 1975, is experiencing guns and vandalism. Both children and teachers feel the need to arm themselves. Your child may no longer be safe at school! Thirty years later and the situation is worsening. In addition, we are now experiencing an epidemic of chronic diseases for which there is seemingly no direct cause and effect. Obesity is assuming a new threat to health. We truly need a framework for health that considers the patient's medical history, background and environment.

Both Democrats and Republicans alike talk about starting programs and cutting programs as though a program exists that will cure our woes. Programs that do answer a need are begun only to be phased out when the money runs out or the party in power changes. However, there is a fundamental flaw in most of these programs—they are built on the deficit model where the applicant must identify and emphasize their inadequacies. They do not address the core of our problems, in fact, they have a negative impact. (e.g., absent husbands and fathers in order to secure welfare checks.) This is clearly outlined by Bronfenbrenner, late professor emeritus at Cornell University in a presentation to television producers and writers on September 18, 1981:

The basic operating principle [is that] those who have problems are to be helped by those who have the needed resources; Lady Bountiful has merely yielded place to the trained professional. The deficit model pervades all types of social agencies, but its distinctive properties are revealed in highest relief in our welfare system. To qualify for help, potential recipients must first prove that they and their families are inadequate—they must do so in writing, a dozen times over, with corroborating documentation, so that there can be little doubt that they, and their children, are in fact the inadequate persons they claim to be. Moreover, our mode of service is categorical, to obtain needed help, potential recipients must first be classified into the types of problems they represent. The only way in which they become whole human beings again is to have enough things wrong. Then they can be defined, and dealt with, as problem children, or, better still for bureaucratic purposes, as multiproblem families.... What is the effect of this model on its intended beneficiaries?... The most salient statistics bearing on the issue are the following: Paralleling the changes in family structure in recent years are time series data reflecting the impaired well-being and development of children as manifested in declining levels of academic performance and rising rates of child homicide, suicide, [and] teenage crime.[7]

In other words, not only are family configurations changing (with resultant negative societal changes), but the data collected show that our government's way of dealing with family problems—through negative labeling—is contributing to society's problems of crime, poor education and declining mental health.

In addition, consider where we are in maternal health: women in all industrialized countries outranking the U.S. in infant mortality (lower death rate) have universal access to prenatal care. Some countries even offer monetary benefits to those who seek care early and consistently. In the United States, on the other hand, only 79 percent of white mothers and 61 percent of black, Puerto Rican, North American and Mexican-American mothers have access to prenatal care.[8]

Moreover, research reported by the Health and Human Services Agency for Health Care Policy and Research[9] clearly shows that, even when programs are available at well-baby clinics and the like, it is the lack of education of the mother that accounts for the gap in visits to the clinic to protect children's health.

Any school psychologist will attest to the many barriers to learning that children bring to school, including vision and hearing problems, cultural differences, low self-concept, weak identity, poor concentration, and language difficulties. All of these difficulties confront overburdened teachers, a part-time school nurse, and a one-day-a-week psychologist (if the school is considered well-staffed).

Where Do We Go From Here?

What is needed is a partnership for children—a coalition of government, industry, health clinics, schools, and parents who would form or reform our institutions in such a way as to PREVENT a major portion of our problems and encourage positive growth.

The difficulty with present social programs is that they address the problem after the fact. We have rising statistics in all the usual human behavioral problems but we fail to direct our efforts to PREVENT them. Of course, not all can be prevented, but a comprehensive effort, together with everyone's understanding of what needs to be changed will eventually accomplish our goal of a free society. Two good examples of preventive action are the reduction of smoking and the raising of our nutritional consciousness. Awareness of the lethality of tobacco and the need for less fat and more vitamins were ideas that did not sell to the American public until they knew the facts and they freely decided to change their behavior. With government and business supporting these concepts, we are slowly becoming successful.

We must apply the same preventive principles to developing our greatest resource—our children—and our efforts must be positive. Our goal as parents is to raise our children to be joyous, creative human beings. Vibrant health, maturity relative to our age, a sense of accomplishment, and the ability to love and be loved are all needed to be fully human. We will always have some rich and some poor with us—economic inequities, pain, and suffering. What we need to learn is the way to develop our human qualities so we can deal with the realities of such difficulties while still retaining our ability to be connected to one another. That can only be done, I believe, if we know ourselves biologically, psychologically, and spiritually. Knowledge helps us to make free (positive) choices. Some of this learning can be accomplished in the classroom but much of it has to be experienced in interaction with other loving human beings.

Strategies For The Future

A comprehensive, preventive plan for integrated health education could be accomplished in several ways. It would require cooperation and national determination but with carefully planned steps and demonstration pilots our goals of a healthy, harmonious community would be gradually reached. The plan would include:

1. Cabinet level National Family Commission

2. Family impact statements issued and nationally distributed for all legislation

3. Access to comprehensive, professionally staffed health services in all schools

4. Extension of such school clinic services to pregnant women and families in the community

5. Integration of health, environmental and occupational information and training into school curriculum

6. Changes in our expectations of teachers and consequent changes in teacher training

7. Agreements with business and professional agencies for apprenticeship and intern experiences

8. Daycare centers affiliated with high schools staffed with professionals and with student interns

9. Family Leave insurance

Ambitious, yes. Doable, yes.

As Dr. Mike Samuels reminds us:

> Being aware of human interconnectedness with the universe, of the relationship among all living systems that transcends the age, sets the stage for a transition from an exploitive to an integrative use of all natural resources.[10]

Natural resources include all of us. We are not separate from the universe—in fact our cooperation with the Earth ensures our survival. Children need to learn a cosmology they can live with. Our world is a fast-changing one with new substances in the atmosphere. Children will need all the information they can get to survive as adults.

Application Of Strategies

In keeping with the cybernetic principle of government, it is my conviction that all pending legislation should carry a 'family well-being impact' statement, comparable to and even beyond, the environmental impact statements that are currently used. Had such an impact statement been considered in drafting welfare and tax laws in the past, many unemployed or marginally employed fathers would not have been driven to leave home so that their 'deserted' families could receive public assistance. Working single mothers could have deducted child-care costs from their tax returns as a business expense. Indeed, I believe that a family well-being impact statement is so important a concept that a cabinet position should be created so that pertinent family research and data can be included along with data from budget, agriculture, labor, etc. in forming policies for the nation. In this time of budget cuts and welfare reforms, there is no family impact statement issued or publicly debated so that real information can trickle down to the man in the street whose life is affected. Only fragments of data and non-informative congressional TV hearings are available. Unbelievably, in this age of information and Internet, the truth of how legislation will affect our lives is still secluded and manipulated behind closed doors.

Once the national stage is set for a comprehensive appreciation of the importance of the family, a comprehensive, wellness-based health curriculum would provide families with information and motive to take responsibility for their health. Dr. William Hittler at the National Institute at Steven's Point, Wisconsin has developed a wellness model that could be both preventative and comprehensive and adaptable for schools.

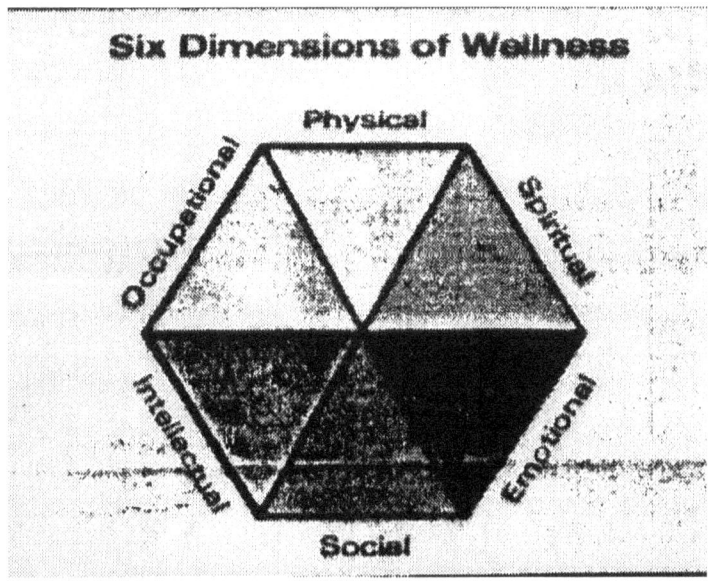

Figure 12-1 Wellness—(Hittler)

Briefly, wellness is a state of being that can be achieved through the balance and integration of diverse aspects of one's life. These aspects (shown above) are identified as the body, mind, spirit, emotions, ambitions, and relationships of an individual.

Wellness is preventative in nature and positive in its goal of a healthy, well-integrated individual. Wellness is dependent on the free choices of the individual which are in turn dependent on how fully informed the individual may be. In practicing wellness, the individual creates a sense of well-being for his/her self, affecting everyone with whom s/he comes in contact. In order to attain this sense of well-being one must set reasonable, individual lifestyle goals and act in a manner which will achieve the goal.

For example, walking has become a favorite preventative health practice that is taking hold in the general population. It is up to the individual to decide whether walking is something that would be personally beneficial and enjoyable and set up a schedule which s/he can adhere to.

As a nation, we are slowly coming to an awareness of how life-style affects an individual's general health. There's evidence that regardless of the behavior changed, the very act of successful change has a positive effect on health by enhancing our self-confidence and sense of control. We gained proof in the reduction of smokers. Suppose we were to adopt the wellness model as a nation? That would mean our health system would need to focus on achieving and maintaining health rather than on identifying and eradicating disease, as worthy as these goals may be. Further, in order to be effective, any such wellness attitudes would have to be communicated to and assimilated within the family, for it is through examples in the home that children learn and develop healthy life habits thus allowing the process to pass on to the next generation.

In *Well Body, Well Earth*, author Samuels makes clear:

> Like radio buoys guarding a ship at sea, disease and health can guide our lives. Steering our course by these signals not only leads to a life relatively free of disease, it can also guide us to the upper limits of personal fulfillment…because of our interconnectedness the fulfillment of any single individual or system ultimately benefits all systems around it. Guided by disease and health,…the living Earth benefits from every person's human fulfillment.[11]

In schools, wellness is best taught according to educator Jerome Bruner's "spiral curriculum" (See Figure 11-5), which requires that the same concepts be reintroduced year after year, but with greater depth and enrichment as the child grows older and is better able to understand.

Each school, public and private, would house or have access to a wellness clinic providing access to the services of a physician (internist/pediatrician), midwife, nurse practitioner, psychologist, and counselors. The size of the school body would determine the number of staff. Ideally, a low pupil-doctor ratio would be maintained. The clinic would provide comprehensive, preventative medical attention for all children attending the school. Since school attendance is mandated, it would mean that no school-aged child would be without health care (in 1994, 10 million Americans under 18 were uninsured) Such broad-based services would identify incipient conditions early. Staff, working as a team, would promote the general categories of wellness, both in classes and on an individual basis. A low annual fee similar to a book fee could be set for each child so that families would be contributing.

Another advantage of the holistic-based wellness clinic is that the stigma of dealing with emotional problems would be reduced, if not eliminated. Since records would be confidential and since psychologists and counselors would be at the same clinic as medical staff, the nature of the services given each child would not readily be evident. In other words, the kid with emotional problems would not be singled out by classmates since all students would visit the clinic regularly.

To provide a nurturing environment outside of school, the clinic would serve a further needed purpose. Any pregnant woman in the neighborhood of the school would be eligible to utilize the school clinic for education, counseling, and medical referral for free obstetrical care. As of now, 25 percent of American women have no health insurance, have to wait in long lines for care, and have no choice in physicians. Often, they see several doctors during their pregnancy, which is hardly reassuring to the mother-to-be. Nor does it promote educational continuity. For these proposed school health services, those who had medical insurance would be encouraged to utilize that method of payment. Families would have access to counseling, and if necessary, would be aided in filling out required forms. Those who did not have insurance would be provided equal services.

Classes for mothers-to-be, which would include education for nutrition, physical and emotional health of mother and baby during pregnancy, and the effect of life-style choices on the growing fetus, would be taught by the clinic's staff. Also affiliated with this health clinic would be a team of maternal aides—a concept already implemented in Japan, Sweden and other parts of Western Europe. These aides would visit the home during the time the mother was taking classes, to encourage the mother to adapt the class information to her individual circumstances. Application of learning is vital for real integration. These aides would become familiar with each woman they visited during pregnancy so that after delivery, regular visits could be made to offer help in caring for the child. It is well-established that a woman's post partum emotional state is important to the well-being of her child and her own health. Support provided at this time is extremely important.

Thereafter, the mother and child (and father, if possible) would make monthly and then bimonthly visits to the wellness clinic until the child was four years of age. This would ensure access to health care for all under-school-aged children as well as valuable education for their parents. Parents would learn about gender identity and sexual development in early childhood. They would become more comfortable passing on what they learned to their children in non-threatening ways, creating a healthier climate for adult sexual behavior.

At the age of four, if Headstart programs were available in that particular neighborhood, the child would be enrolled while retaining access to the services of the school clinic. If kindergarten was the child's first school experience, continuing medical care would be received without a break. In other words, children would receive care from the time they were in their mother's womb until they graduated from high school. From first through eighth grades, those with serious illnesses diagnosed at the clinic would be referred to the local hospital; however, a small infirmary would be available to care for temporary illness (colds, etc.) for children whose parents were not available to them during the day. Bon Secour, a hospital in Florida, offers this type of care for sick children of working parents. While attending high school, students would be seen regularly during the year, or as necessary upon request. Again, after diagnosis, referrals for serious cases would be made to the appropriate agency.

From a practical perspective, such a system would help in early identification of those children needing help of some kind. For very young children, the maternal aides would act as a liaison with the family to determine any existing problems that the child might not be able or willing to verbalize. The appropriate staff expert could then pursue the matter further.

Let's see how it would work:

Johnny Smith is 6 years old and lives on Green Street in a so-so neighborhood. He will register in the first grade this fall. At P.S.16 where Johnny will go to school, there is a wellness clinic staffed by a physician, midwife, nurse practitioner, psychologist, counselor, and maternal aides. The size of the staff provides a low pupil-staff ratio so that each child will receive sufficient attention.

As he entered school, a free medical examination found that Johnny had a hearing problem. He was referred to a community audiologist for a hearing evaluation and possible hearing aid. It was also discovered by the psychologist that Johnny hated his younger sister because she was taking all of his mother's attention. A visit to the home by the nurse practitioner revealed that Johnny's mother (Connie) had a three-year-old daughter (Maria) with cerebral palsy and was also five months pregnant. Connie had no doctor nor had she been examined or counseled since the beginning of her pregnancy.

The nurse practitioner was able to refer Maria to the clinic physician with her recommendations as well as giving Connie a suitable referral to a daycare situation for disabled children. She was also able to persuade Connie to attend the health classes at school provided by the wellness clinic medical staff. A maternal aide was assigned to the family for the sake of continuity of care and to help Connie implement the information that she learned in class. Counseling services were available as needed.

Thus we have a potentially violent situation prevented, i.e. a growing boy able to devote his energy to learning rather than dissipating it in anger at his sister or in frustration from a hearing impairment. We have two physical dysfunctions cared for and two community resources appropriately utilized. Further, and probably most important, a pregnant mother is being educated so as to prevent possible birth defects or malnutrition in the developing child. What Connie learns about nutrition will help the whole family.

This is only one example of how the school-health clinic partnership would benefit the whole community. The clinic provides the services, the school provides the consumers who benefit in both health and education. Community cohesiveness would be developed as the health patterns of that particular neighborhood became better known and better served. An environment of trust would ensue, as parents began to see the results with their children and in the family.

These continuing health services would also provide a complete health care history for each child. Consider the data that could be used as a basis for health research! Parents would also be encouraged to keep a similar record, and could be provided with a book for appropriate entries.

In summary, this preventative approach would attempt to meld community (neighborhood-based) health care with the school system. The health care in effect prior to school attendance would have outreach components to address the needs of pregnant woman, parents, infants, and toddlers. It would help to insure the child's readiness to enter school without barriers to learning. This model could be expanded or reduced according to the needs of the specific locales.

A community clinic approach has been in existence since 1897. According to the Web site, www.queenscarefamilyclinics.org, the Franciscans founded a clinic to care for the abandoned and neglected children of Los Angeles. In 1930 the Franciscan Sisters of the Sacred Heart made room for the small clinic in Queen of Angels Hospital. In 1998 Arthur Barrin and J.J.. Brandlin, former Trustees of the Queen of Angels Hollywood Presbyterian Medical Center, formed Queens Care, a unique corporation that is both a direct provider and a dispenser of grants to local non-profit agencies. Direct provider services include dental and vision, providing for 35,000 students and 7000 pairs of glasses. Two vans serviced 50,000 school children's toothaches.

The problems posed by family mobility and rapidly changing neighborhoods could be overcome—or at least minimized—with the use of progressive electronic communication systems.

Does this sound way out? Remember, we have an emergency situation! We are twenty-fifth in infant mortality among industrial nations. Successful reproduction is more than a safe delivery. It is the physiological, neurological, psychological and social development of that infant as a healthy member of society. We must change our education and health service delivery to safeguard the next generation. The cost of prevention is much lower—so much lower as not to be compared with the cost of dysfunction.

Strategies 5, 6 And 7

Needless to say, such a comprehensive approach to health education would require integration into the context of the regular school curriculum. Ideally, with health monitoring taking place from the womb to the beginning of school, plus the education of families as to healthful lifestyles, the child would have absorbed on a limited level some idea of the importance of health. What would naturally follow, then, is that the child would be taught the reasons why this is important. Their intellectual development would include a scientifically based knowledge of their bodies and how the care of it is inextricably connected to the environment.

The health based educational system would be taught in tandem with environmental information. Children would learn that they are part of the life energy force that forms our earth. Children can be taught that their behavior is important to their own health, the health of their community and to the environment of the earth as a whole. This would be information available to all children—not compromised by divisive systems of Medicaid, welfare, ethnic origin or public/private funding. Each child would be regarded as a precious responsibility to develop into a healthy, well-integrated adult. Not only for the sake of the child but for all of us who inhabit the earth. What a background for the future citizens of our global world. What an example for other countries to follow! This would truly be a new, world order—a healthy one!

For example, how exciting for a child in first grade to be given a model of an individual cell to examine, to be taught that this is how his body began. To learn that each cell contains directions on how it should develop—e.g., eyes, ears, etc. He would have a sense of his own importance, gaining a respect for his body as something to be cared for. Such a beginning would help him/her to understand there is an underlying principle of order in human life. Then he could be helped to understand that the earth began from a similar primitive cell and how it has evolved.

The child would gain a beginning vision of what Dr. Mike Samuels states so clearly in his book, *Well Body, Well Earth*:

> Everything in the universe is now built from the same elementary particles, those being electrons, protons and neutrons. These 3 basic building blocks have combined and recombined in various patterns over the ages to become everything in and on the earth.... Since we can trace our own beginnings to these universal, elementary particles, it became obvious that we are all kin.... We humans are not separate or impermeable. On the contrary, it is our permeability and our kinship through the elementary particles that we share with the universe that makes our lives possible.[12]

In keeping with Dr. Bruner's cyclical concept of education (see Figure 11-5), in the second year, the child might learn how the cell needs nourishment; how the mother provides nourishment and loving environment. Further, how the earth needs nourishment and that we provide that nourishing environment by our habits. As the child progresses, s/he learns the importance of good food and how the earth provides it. Gradually, s/he is taught to expect Dr. Hansell's seven essentials for life while relating the securing of them to the preservation of our earth, and to the health of their bodies. Such a curriculum, developed by experts of course, would develop skills for personal satisfaction and independence so important to the child's vulnerable emotional health.

By the time children reach the fifth grade, their bodies have already begun to undergo the changes of puberty, and they are very much in need of relevant information. Their growing bodies and developing personalities are the first order of business for them. We should capitalize on this interest. When I was in sixth grade, a very forward-looking teacher taught us physiology. We learned about veins, arteries, the function of the heart, the need for oxygen, etc. I have never forgotten the marvels opened to my mind. Unfortunately, what was missing was an explanation of the reproductive system. Such instruction was unheard of at the time.

Recently, on Public Television, I was fortunate to view a program prepared by the Children's Television Workshop.[13] It was an excellent presentation of the physical needs and uses of our bodies and the feelings and fears that surround the beginning years of adolescence. What I felt was unfortunate was the choice of its title, *Sex Education*. Since society's emphasis is generally on genital sex, I would have preferred a title such as *Life-styles and Your Sexuality*. This would have been a more comprehensive title that would have conveyed some sense of individual responsibility. Nonetheless, the material covered was excellent and was presented well.

Oprah Winfrey and her male co-host, facilitating a group of teen-agers, conveyed very skillfully that bodily changes and sexual urges are normal, healthy and need to be acknowledged, not denied. The real purpose of this sexual development—to help the teen-ager grow to healthy maturity when they could choose to raise a family—was emphasized rather than negative behavior. However consequences of too early sexual activity were made clear. We need more of this type of instruction.

Parents should have access to such school programs thus giving them some understanding of and input into what information would be presented to their children. Ideally, parents would have kept pace with their children's sexual development with frank discussions, but so often, parents either cannot or will not do so.

If we would present genital or erotic sex positively, but as only one facet of sexuality to be used only with love and commitment, I believe that more boys and girls would have a greater sense of responsibility about their behavior.

What is usually taught is exactly the opposite—how to enjoy the pleasure of erotic sex without "getting caught" or having to be committed to a relationship. Fourth graders are taught about venereal disease and AIDS. Teen-agers actually believe the advertisers of condoms as safe sex, with the same idea often promoted by school authorities. The reasoning is "the kids will be sexually active anyway, so let's teach them how to do it responsibly."

The truth of the matter is that were these youngsters' self-esteem not damaged and had they experienced a responsible adult support system that challenged their talents and demanded individual responsible choices, they would not have to express their need for approval, affirmation and love with inappropriate sexual behavior. Such skills as decision-making, communication skills, conflict resolution, how to be a friend, gender differences, and what to expect of a relationship are all part of the understanding of sexuality to which each child is entitled.

In addition to these skills, the sixth grade to eighth grade curriculum would ideally include coping skills, or, if you will, survival skills. Both boys and girls would learn how to nourish themselves, cook, shop, maintain their own hygiene and clothing, use tools, and do routine home maintenance. Skills that working parents no longer have time to teach their children. As it stands now, these skills are included in programs for teen-agers not expected to go beyond vocational school. What I am advocating is an effort to help each individual student to develop as independently as possible in practical everyday coping, given their age and experience.

In high school, driver education would be extended to include how to care for a car and what is involved to finance one. Such skills would not only enhance their self-esteem and help build an attitude of responsibility but would prepare them for the world of work. There is nothing that helps confidence as much as being able to cope independently.

As a natural follow-up, internships and apprenticeships could be arranged, following the German plan of hands-on teaching. In Germany, students as young as thirteen years of age are apprenticed in factories and industry as part of their education. This format could be extended, as various kinds of businesses cooperated, for engineers, business practices, teachers, medical workers—whatever would be the student's interest.

Such a comprehensive curriculum would help students to reach the goals of wellness, esteem for self and others, responsibility and self-discipline. It would lessen the tedium of strictly verbal instruction in the classroom where instead lively discussions and questions based on the student's hands-on experiences could take place. It would assist students in their choice of satisfactory life goals (job-satisfaction is part of health and wellness). Thus the wellness goals of intellectual, social and occupational information would be accomplished. Students would, through their experiences, develop their own system of meaning. The physical, psychological and spiritual aspects of development would be supported.

Such a curriculum would teach students that patriotism is not giving oneself in battle so much as it is preparing oneself for life so that one can contribute to making a peaceful community in a manner based on one's own unique talents.

It cannot be stressed enough that individuals require emotional security gained by being competent masters at solving daily problems. As Valerius Geist, states that: "without any control over environment comes despair, deep depression, then disease and finally death. Depression is a disease of our time!"[14]

Parental Involvement

It is essential that parents cooperate with this comprehensive wellness curriculum. With both parents at work, there is little time and energy left to do much. However, it is essential—so we must find a way. The maternal aide from these school clinics would be one method. They would prevent those students of uncooperative parents from falling through the cracks of home and school. As parents get to trust what the schools are doing, when they see the benefits in their own children, they may become willing to sacrifice their precious time to cooperate. However, school authorities must insure parental participation by requiring parents to be present for their child's health consultation every semester. Hopefully the staff-parent relationship would be a harmonious one, geared solely to the healthy development of the child. Also, teaching parenting within the curriculum would make parenting more important to adolescent students while training them to become parents.

A good example of such a training course is presently being tried in 36 New York City schools. Initiated by Lou Howart, teacher at The High School of the Humanities, and developed with Dr. Margaret Kind, psychiatrist at Metropolitan Hospital, the course starts with pre-natal care and includes many of the ideas contained in this book.

1. Infancy—Emotional social development, including attachment, separation-individuation, separation anxiety, stranger anxiety
2. Toddler (age 1-3)—Intellectual and language development, including the need for parental stimulation, parental development and the authority stage.

Howart's main goal in teaching this class is to "cut down on physical and mental abuse (of children) and to prevent teenage pregnancy."[15]

Besides teaching in the classroom, there is a further hands-on method. It has always been a dream of mine to locate daycare facilities near high schools so that teenagers could be apprenticed there and experience, first-hand, the needs of children in preparation for their own parenting experience. Such practice would not only benefit the growing young adult but would also provide an excellent environment for the little ones who are separated from their parents for long hours. Kids relate well to each other…learning easily from one another.

In parenting classes such as that of Professor Howart, the student would learn the fundamentals underlying understanding an infant and then spend hands on time learning the nitty gritty practice. In addition to being apprentices in the daycare center, students could choose to be apprentices at the health clinic. They would learn how medical clinics are run, what nurses do, what it is to see others suffer, how to help them with kindness. Contact with any art or science, especially with a cooperative professional, inspires young people to create similar goals for themselves. It helps to give focus to their learning when they see what can be accomplished with knowledge. Questions born of this kind of experience could be confronted and debated in the classroom, helping the individual student to integrate his own knowledge.

Outline For Change

In order to put such a curriculum into practice, a change in attitude on the national level concerning the value of education must take place. The influence of high value given to education in the home cannot be overemphasized. How both interact is interestingly demonstrated by research done over a 10-year period beginning in 1980.

A cross-cultural study conducted by Dr. Harold Stevenson was reported in the December 1992 issue of Scientific American.[16] Dr. Stevenson compared American schools with those in East Asian countries. His methodology and specific reports cannot be reproduced here, but briefly, he found that school children in Asia performed better academically than those in the United States. Further, they enjoyed going to school for longer hours! Some of the reasons for the differences included more recess periods, using more real objects for close observation rather than verbal instruction, the value assigned to education by parents, and surprisingly, the extensive amount of attention the teachers gave the children.

Teachers in the United States are often held responsible for six classes per day, taught in isolation. Their preparation work is mostly done on their own time in the evening when they are tired. By contrast, Asian teachers only teach about three hours a day and use the rest of the day for class preparation and consulting with colleagues about better ways to present materials to students. What a boon this system would be to overworked American teachers.

Dr. Stevensen describes Asian teachers:

> Asian teachers can be described best as well-informed well-prepared guides. They do not see themselves primarily as dispensers of information and arbiter of what is correct but rather as persons responsible for guiding students skillfully through the material.[17]

Brief periods of seatwork are interspersed throughout the class time to practice what has just been learned, in contrast to the lengthy periods of seatwork that are the norm in American schools. Immediate feedback, which is essential for learning, is then given to the students on the seat work performed. For how else does a child know that he or she understands the concept presented?

It would seem that Asian schools (and Montessori schools as well) are built on a respect for the unfolding of the unique individual. That respect begins with

1. Care in the womb
2. Fostering connectedness and neurologic development
3. Placing children first in importance without losing our adult identity
4. Allowing children to grow at their own pace, utilizing their uniqueness instead of placing them in categories and boxes.

Another good example of hands-on teaching is the American medical schools, considered to be the best in the world. After the first year, medical students live, study and practice in hospitals with live patients. Such responsibility, combined with learning, is of true educational value.

There is no doubt that these educational principles, fostered in a comprehensive health-integrated educational system, implemented on a national basis, would change our school system for the better. But how will parents have time for this change if both are working?

Family Supportive Strategies

In this present climate of feminism, there is controversy over who should stay home with the newborn. Mom or Dad? It is well to remember that a 9-month old relationship has at birth already been established between mother and baby. For optimum development of both mother and baby, they should be together until the infant's identity is established. During this time, they both need full support of the father. This is a critical period in the development of family cohesiveness and can be and often is a period of strain on family relationships.

Leaving the gender issue aside for the moment, how can family leave be accomplished in this day and age of two-wage-earner parents? How can family leave be established with fairness to employer, employee, parents, and children? How can freedom of choice be protected while protecting the right of the child to optimal growth?

It Can Be Done!

First, as I have said at several points in this book, society must change its attitude. Care of infants and children is vitally important WORK, work equal to any in the marketplace and should have the same benefits. Mothers are prime educators. If they have failed in this role, one reason is because society has always felt education was wasted on girls who would soon be married. Presently, society views education of women only vital for work in the marketplace.

Second, instead of women apologizing for being at home, they should be supported and educated to the same degree as any teacher by all of society. They are certainly entitled to the right of choice. An excellent book, *Home by Choice*, written by Brenda Hunter (1991) would enlighten many mothers.

Third, we must find an economic solution to family leave. I would like to offer a plan for subsidizing family leave via a channel similar to that established for unemployment insurance. In essence, it would provide for the gap in benefit to homemakers who are denied unemployment benefits when they leave work voluntarily because of pregnancy. Remember, care of children is WORK. Using the same administration mechanism now in place for unemployment insurance, everyone—employer and employee alike—would pay into a family leave insurance fund. This would be a small percentage of the total wage (possibly 2 percent). The rationale for everyone contributing is that the community at large would benefit. Such a fund could be drawn upon by a first-time mother who was six months into her pregnancy (depending on health factors) until approximately three years after the birth of her child. She would draw a weekly sum of family leave insurance, commensurate with (in proportion to) her former wages. She would become eligible for such support by securing prenatal care and attending some type of training session to increase her knowledge of how to care for the baby. Subsequent births would require the same eligibility criteria.

The amount of family insurance paid would be much less than the gross amount of the prevailing wage. However, when the cost of daycare, clothes, transportation, lunches and taxes are deducted from the gross wage, the difference between the amount of wages, and the amount of insurance would be small indeed.

Such a supportive plan would underscore society's view of responsible parenthood in marriage and would provide an incentive for high school graduates to train for the world of work if they wish to benefit from the plan. Such a plan could conceivably influence the number of children born out of wedlock by providing an incentive to work before marriage in order to become eligible. Would an employer hold a job for such women who took advantage of the plan? That would depend on the individual circumstances and the type of job. Certainly the same or comparable work could be made available.

How would such a plan affect the employer's business? Taking three years leave would be inconvenient to be sure, but not incapacitating. Training a substitute employee, who would be hired with that understanding, could be accomplished by the departing mother. She could be on call for a month to answer any questions. Perhaps, women could team work a job to provide a continuous workforce.

Not everyone would choose to stay home. Not all mothers would avail themselves of this plan. My own personal solution to the problem of early child care was not to work until after our children were two years old and then to work part time for the next two or three years, working my hours around my husband's schedule. I happened to be fortunate in that my employer was flexible. There are other means of providing for early childcare by the mother. The U.S. Bureau of Labor Statistics claims that the average American changes jobs every three years and shifts careers about every six years. It is feasible to change jobs or careers to suit the demands of child care rather than regulate the care of the child to jobs or careers. Again, that would, however, require national commitment to the importance of childcare.

Another means of coping with this problem is flextime. With the cooperation of business, this is a system whereby mother and father arrange their work schedules so that one or the other is with the child.

Another option is working at home. With the proliferation of computers and fax machines, it is realistically possible to increase the number of home workers. One young attorney worked at home after her infant was born and her leave was up and returned to work six months later—to her former position.

There has been some discussion of both men and women working three-fourths time—a thirty-two hour week instead of the forty, sixty, or eighty hours worked by some professionals (this has already been adopted in some places in Europe). A shorter work week would leave more time for family activities and community involvement. It would also provide additional jobs for the unemployed. In our modern culture, too much noise and overcrowding plus a lack of control over one's life creates a great deal of stress. Perhaps we should emulate earlier civilizations who were less stressed and who allotted much more time for family and community leisure.

Many creative solutions are possible if we begin with the premise that child care, especially infant care, is a number one priority. If one has a child, the most important work one can do is to accept the responsibility of bringing that child to his or her optimal level of development. By doing so, you serve society, yourself, and your child. With societal help, career paths, while important, can be made to bend to accommodate our children. For too long, we in America have put industry first and children second.

If your choice is not to have a child, then your obligation is to contribute to a family leave fund for others who choose to have children. That is a societal obligation, the same as caring for the elderly. In addition, you are in a unique position to be an aunt, uncle, or relative of some degree to those children you know who would benefit from your love. This also is a role that is unrecognized by society for its degree of importance.

On Making Human Beings Human

Bronfenbrenner, the world renowned sociologist, sets out four propositions that are essential for human growth for "making human beings human."[18]

1. In order to develop normally, a child needs the enduring irrational involvement of one or more adults in care and joint activity with the child.... Someone has to be there, and to be doing something—not alone, but together with the child.

2. The developmental impact of emotionally involved care and joint activity with the child is enhanced by the participation of adults of both sexes in the process.

3. The developmental potential of a setting depends upon the extent to which third parties present support (or undermine) the activities of those actually engaged in interaction with the child.

4. The involvement of one or more adults in care and joint activity in support of child rearing requires public policies and practices that provide opportunity, status, resources, encouragement, example, stability and above all, time for parenthood, primarily by parents but also by other adults in the child's environment, both within and outside the home.

When asked what was the age of the child to whom he was referring, Bronfenbrenner said it was debatable but he thought anyone under the age of eighty-nine! Underscoring the fact that we never outgrow the need to be connected and loved.

This well-respected sociologist further pointed out that an examination of the principles speak to the human condition also:

> As human biologists remind us—one of the distinguishing features of the species Homo Sapiens is that we are social animals. Sooner or later—and in between—we need each other. To give recognition to this reality in our four propositions, one has only to substitute the words "human being" for "child" and replace "parent" with "relatives, friends and neighbors."

Based on an analysis of the available research evidence, these four propositions describe critical features of the ecology that are conducive to making human beings human.[19]

Personal decisions with regard to our own sexuality are important not only for the individual but also the community at large. Ignorance and denial of our sexuality, promiscuity and commercialization of sex have brought disease and chaos in our society. We must be alert to our natural pathways to mature sexuality, mindful of its critical periods and what influences its development. In recognizing our sexuality, we must begin with the assumption that men and women are different—physically, psychologically and spiritually. These differences have nothing to do with equality—in fact our commonality lies in the recognition of these differences.

Interaction between the sexes strongly influences their own sexual identity as well as those of our children. Unfortunately, recognition of this fact will take a long time for each individual has to form core beliefs for him or herself before our culture will fully recognize an acceptable pattern of sexual behavior. We have strayed far from the innate nature of our being. Insofar as our beliefs and values influence the way we vote, the stands we take on community issues and the way we treat others around us, it is important to determine whether the assumptions underlying our current values are accurate.

As I see it, we need to consciously choose family-sustainable, societal structures that support the welfare of our children, and we must do it now. To do less is to risk our survival. I have suggested plans for comprehensive, health-education integration, high school daycare centers, and family leave insurance. In these, I believe lie the beginnings of our new world order. What will you add to these solutions?

In brief…

❖ The needs of children are paramount to the ordered growth of society.

❖ Care of our physical bodies, development of emotional sensitivity, and recognition of the larger aspects of our spirituality, need to be supported by the rules laid down by our society.

❖ Education can be optimally assimilated only by a child who is healthy and has a strong emotional tie to someone.

❖ Health care from conception to death is of prime importance in maintaining our global position in the new order.

❖ Building strong, self-reliant, sexually mature youth is our nation's greatest asset—economic or otherwise.

❖ Individuals with a developed sense of their lovability, sexual identity, and autonomy seek lives with meaning that include respect for self and others. They, for the most part, are at peace. Peaceful individuals engender a peaceful society.

CHAPTER 12—EndNotes

1   Erikson, Erik, H., *Identity and the Life Cycle*, International University Press, New York, N. Y. 1959,1980

2   Sykes, Charles J., *A Nation of Victims, The Decay of the American Character*, St. Martin's Press, New York, NY 1992

3   Hansell, Norris, M.D., *The Person in Distress*, Behavioral Publications, Inc., Human Science Press, New York, NY 1976

4   Hewlitt, Sylvia Ann, *When the Bough Breaks, The Cost of Neglecting Our Children*, Harper & Co., New York, NY 1991

5   Beasley, Joseph D. M.D., *The Betrayal of Health*, Times Book (Random House Incorporated) New York, 1991

6   Geist, Valerius. *Children's Initiative, Synopsis of Interim Findings* Child Abuse Center, Report from SCAA, 1 Columbia Place, Albany, N.Y.,

7   Bronfenbrenner, Urie, "New Images of Children", Winter 1982, *Families & American Television & Children*, Fall, 1981

8   Karta, Diane, "Infant Mortality, Japan Ranks First", *Mothering Magazine*, Vol. 62, Winter 1992, Santa Fe, New Mexico

9   Samuels, Mike, M.D. and Nancy Samuels, *The Well Baby Book*, Summit Books, Simon & Schuster, New York, N.Y., 1979

10 Ibid

11 Samuels, op cit

12 Samuels, op cit

13 Silverstone, Robert, Dr., and Rhonda Wise, "What Kids Want To Know About", *Children's Television Workshop*, Lincoln Place, New York, NY—shown Channel 17 (Buffalo, NY) 5/13/92

14 Geist, Valerius, op cit

15 Medzian, Myriam, *Boys Will Be Boys*, Doubleday, New York, NY, 1991

16 Stevenson, Harold W., "Learning from Asian Schools", *Scientific American*, December, 1992

17 Ibid

18 Bronfenbrenner, Urie, op cit

19 Ibid

Bibliography

Books

Arraj, James, *St. John of the Cross and Dr. C. G. Jung*, Inner Growth Books, Chiloquin, Ohio, 1986

Beasley, Joseph D. M.D., *The Betrayal of Health*, Times Book (Random House Incorporated) New York, 1991

Bell, Alan, P. Weinberg and S.K. Hammersmith, *Sexual Preference: It's Development in Men and Women.* Indiana University Press, Bloomington, Ind., 1988

Bodanis, David, *The Body Book: A Fantastic Voyage to the World Within* 1984

Borysenko, Joan, *Guilt is the Teacher, Love is the Lesson*, Warner Books, New York, N.Y., 1990

Buscaglia, Leo T., *Personhood*, Chas. Block, Inc., Tharafare, N. Y., 1978

Callwood, June, *Emotions, What They Are and How They Affect Us*, Doubleday & Co., New York, N.Y., 1986

Caplan, Gerard, *Principles of Preventive Psychiatry*, Basic Books, New York, N.Y., 1964

Carroll, James, *Constantine's Sword*, Paulist Press, New York, NY, 2001.

Coles, Robert, M. D., *Spiritual Life of Children*, Houghton, Mifflin, New York, N.Y., 1990

Coles, Robert, *The Youngest Parents: Teenage Pregnancy As It Shapes Lives*, New York: Center for Documentary Studies in association with WW Norton & Company, New York & London, 1997

de Castellijo, Irene Claremont, M.D., *Knowing Women*, Harper Colophon Books, Harper & Row, New York, NY, 1974 de Chardin, Teilhard, *The Evolution of Chastity, Toward the Future*, (R.Hague, E. Traus), Harcourt, Brace, Jovanvich, New York, N.Y., 1975

Dominion, Jack, *Affirming the Human Personality*, Darton, Longman & Todd, Ltd, London, 1975

Erikson, Erik, *Identity and the Life Cycle*, W.W. Norton & Co., New York, N.Y., 1959, l980, 1994

Flanagan, Geraldine Lux, *The First Nine Months of Life*, Simon & Schuster, 2nd Edition, New York, NY. 1982

Fromm, Eric, *Heart of Man, Its Genius for Good and Evil*, Harper & Row, New York, N.Y., 1964

Giffen, Mary, M.D., with Carol Felsenthal, *A Cry for Help*, Doubleday & Co., Garden City, New York, 1983

Gilder, George, *Sexual Suicide*, NY Quadrangle, NY Times Book Co, 1973

Hansell, Norris, M. D., *The Person in Distress*, Behavioral Publications, Inc., Human Science Press, New York, NY 1976

Hastings, Arthur C. PhD, et al, *Health for the Whole Person*, Bantum Books, New York, Toronto, London, l976

Helfer, Roy, M.D., *Childhood Comes First, A childhood Crash Course for Adults*, Self-published, East Lansing, Mich. 48823, 1978

Herschkowitz, M.D, Norbert. and Elinore Chapman Herschkowitz, *A Good Start in Life: Understanding Your Child's Brain and Behavior*, Joseph Henry Press, Washington, D.C., 2002

Hewlitt, Sylvia Ann, *When the Bough Breaks, The Cost of Neglecting Our Children*, Harper & Co., New York, NY 1991

Hora, Thomas. *Dialogues in Metapsychiatry*, Seabury Press, New York, N.Y., l975

Hutchinson, Michael, *The Anatomy of Sex and Power, An Investigation of Mind-Body Politics*, Marrow Publishing Co., New York, N.Y., 1990

Hunter, Brenda, *Home by Choice : Raising Emotionally Secure Children in an Insecure World*, Multnomah Publishing Co., Sisters, Oregon1991

Jourard, Sidney, M., *The Transparent Self*, Von Nostrand Reinhold Co., Inc., Florida, l971, revised edition

Joyce, Robert and Mary, *New Dimensions in Sexual Love*. St. John's University Press. Collegeville, MN. 1970

Keen, Sam, *Fire in the Belly—On Being a Man*, Bantam Books, New York, N. Y., 1991

Kinsey, A.C., et al, *Sexual Behavior in the Human Female*, Indiana University Press, Bloomington, IN, l953, 1998.

Kirkpatrick, Wm., Phd., *Identity and Intimacy*, Dell Publishing Co., New York, N.Y., 1964

Leight, Lynn, *Raising Sexually Healthy Children*, Rawson Associates, New York, N.Y., l988

Lepp, Ignace, *The Psychology of Loving*, Helicon, Baltimore, MD, 1963

Lewontin, Richard, *Human Diversity*, Scientific American Library, W.H. Freeman & Co., New York, NY, 1982

Liley, M.M.I., M.D., as cited by Schwartz, *The World of the Unborn*, Marek Publishers, New York, NY l980

Lynn, David B., *The Father, His Role in Child Development*, Brook/Cole Publishing Co., Monterey, CA., 1974

Maguire, Jack and the Philip Leif Group, Inc., *Care and Feeding of the Brain*, Doubleday, New York, NY 1990

Mahler, Margaret, *The Psychological Birth of the Human Infant*, Basic Books, Inc., 1973

Masters, Wm, Johnson, Virginia E., Kolodny, Robert, *Masters & Johnson on Sex and Human Loving*, Little, Brown & Co., Boston/Toronto, 1982/85/86

Medzian, Myriam, *Boys Will be Boys: Breaking the Link between Masculinity and Violence*. New York: Anchor Books, 1991

Michaelmore, Susan, *Sexual Reproduction*, Eyre & Soituswode, Ltd, (England) 1964. The American Museum of Natural History by the Natural Free Press, New York, NY

Moore, Keith L., *The Developing Human, Clinically Oriented Embryology*, Saunders Publishing Co., New York, NY 4th edition, 1988

Moore, Allen J. *The Young Adult Generation: A Perspective on the Future.* New York: Abingdon Press. 1969. Multicultural Resource and Research Center. School of Theology, Claremont, California

Moore, Thomas, *Original Self,* Harper-Collins, NY, NY 2000

Money, John, *Man, Woman, Boy, Girl,* John Hopkins University Press, Baltimore, Md., 1973

Montagu, Ashley, M. D., *Prenatal Influences,* Charles C. Thomas, Springfield, Ill., 1962

Montessori, Maria, *The Child in the Family,* Translated by Nancy Rockmore Cirillo, Henry Regenery Co., Chicago, Ill., 1970

Newton, Niles, M. D., *The Family Book of Child Care,* Harper & Brothers Publishers, New York, N. Y., 1957

Noble, Elizabeth, *Primal Connections,* Simon & Schuster, New York, NY, 1993

Odent, Michael, *Primal Health: A Blueprint for Our Survival,* London Century, 1986

Peerbolte, Lietaert, M., *Prenatal Dynamics,* Leyden, Netherlands, 1954

Prescott, J.W., *Affectional Bonding for the Prevention of Violent Behavior, Neurobiological, Psychological, and Religious/Spiritual Determinants, In Violent Behavior, Vol. 1: Assessment and Intervention* (Hertzberg L.J.etal), OMA Publishing Corp., New York, NY, 1990

Remen, Naomi Rachel, *Kitchen Table Wisdom, Stories That Heal.* Riverhead Books, New York, 1996.

Ribble, Margaret A., M.D., *The Rights of Infants,* Columbia University Press, New York, N.Y., 1943, 13th printing 1957, 1980.

Ricklefs, Robert E., and Finch, Caleb E., *Aging, A Natural History,* Scientific American Library, W.N. Freeman, New York, N. Y., 1995

Rosen, Mortimer, M.D. and Rosen, Lynn, EDD., *In the Beginning: Your Baby's Brain Before Birth,* Plume Book, New Amsterdam Library, New York, N.Y., 1975

Samuels, Mike, M.D. and Nancy Samuels, *The Well Baby Book,* Summit Books, Simon & Schuster, New York, N.Y., 1979

Schwartz, Leni, *The World of the Unborn* Richard Publishers, New York, NY, l980

Silber, Sherman, J., *The Male from Infancy to Old Age*, Charles Scribner, Inc., New York, N. Y., l981

Sorenson, Robert C., *Adolescent Sexuality in Contemporary America*, World Publishing Co., New York, NY, 1973

Stein, Sara, *The Body Book*, Workman Publishing, New York, NY 1992

Stoller, Robert G. *Sex and Gender; On the Development of Masculinity and Femininity*, Science House, New York, NY, 1968

Sykes, Charles J., *A Nation of Victims, The Decay of the American Character*, St. Martin's Press, New York, NY 1992

The Diagram Group, *The Brain, A User's Manual*, Berkeley Publishing Co., New York, N.Y. 1984

Unwin, John, *Sex and Culture*, Oxford U Press, l934, London, England.

Vanier, Jean, *Male and Female, He Created Them*, Paulist Press, Mahwah, New York, N. Y., l984, 85 and l989

Verny, Thomas, M.D., with John Kelly, *The Secret Life of the Unborn*, Summit Books, Division of Simon & Schuster, New York, N.Y., l981

Watts, Alan, *Nature, Man and Woman*, Pantheon Press, New York, New York, l958

West, Melissa Gayle, *If Only I were a Better Mother*, Stillpoint Publishing, Walpole, N.H. 1992

Wolf, Anna, W.M., *The Parents' Manual*, Simon & Schuster, Popular Library Edition, New York, N.Y., 1951

Periodicals

Bronfenbrenner, Urie, "New Images of Children", Winter 1982, "Families & American Television & Children, Fall, 1981

Crews, David, *"Animal Sexuality"*, Scientific American, January 1994, pp. 109-114

Evans, Mari, Maryknoll, July l981—p.33

Fachelmann, Kathy A., "Motherhood and Cancer", Science News, Vol. 142, p.298, October 31, l992

Ferreira, Anthony, J., M.D., "Emotional Factors in Prenatal Environment", Journal of Nervous and Mental Disease, Vol. 141, No. 1, 1965

Glasser, William, M.D., *The Ego, Your Bridge to the World*, from "Blueprint for Health", Blue Cross Association, Vol 20, No. 3, Chicago, Ill, 1960

Hitz, R., Driscoll A, "Praise or Encouragement New insights into Praise: Implications of Early Childhood Teachers" *Young Children*, July 1988

Karta, Diane, "Infant Mortality, Japan Ranks First", Mothering Magazine, Vol. 62, Winter 1992, Santa Fe, New Mexico

Keating, Thomas, "Contemplative Spirituality and Sexuality", Contemplative Outreach News, Vol. 7, Fall, l993

Keniston, Kenneth, "Moral and Ethics", The American Scholar, l965, vol. 34, p.628

McEwen, Bruce, Rockefeller Institute, New York, N.Y., 1992, "U.S News and World Report", 8/8/88

Mulinare, Dr. Joseph, "Readers Digest" April 1989, p.124—"Prevention Magazine" March 1990, pp127-128

Needleman, Jacob, "Questions of the Heart", *Noetic Science Review*, No. 26, Summer, l993, p.5. Sausalito, CA

Nilsson, Linnert, "The Worlds Within Our Bodies", *Life Magazine*, January 1970.

Rupp, Joyce, OSM, *The Dance of Life*, St. Anthony Messenger, May 2002, p 36

Schatz, Carla J., "The Developing Brian", Scientific American, P. 60, September, 1992

Sommers, S., "Emotionally reconsidered, The role of cognition in emotional responsiveness", Journal of Personality and Social Psychology, Vol. 41, p.560, 1981

Sontag, Lester W., "War and the Fetal Maternal Relationship", Marriage and Family Living 6, pp. 1-5, 1944

Sontag, Lester W., "Implications of Fetal Behavior and Environment for Adult Personality", *Annals of New York Academy of Sciences*, pp.782-786, February 1966

Stevenson, Harold W., "Learning from Asian Schools", *Scientific American*, December, 1992

Stott, Dennis, *Follow-up study from Birth of Effects of Prenatal Stress*, Developmental Medicine, Child Neurology, vol. 15, pp. 770-787, London, England, l973

Swanson, John, NCCMHC, "Sexism Strikes Men", American Counselor, Fall, l992, Vol 1, #4

The Journal Of Pediatrics, cited in Vegetarian Times, August 1991, pp.22,24

Newspaper Articles

Dr. Robert N. Hoover, director of Epidemiology and Biostatistics program at National Cancer Institute in Bethesda, Md., Los Angeles Times, 7/13/00

AP News Report, Sun Herald, Orlando, FL 3/14/1998

Julie Samuels, National Institute of Justice Survey with Center for Disease Control, AP report 7/14/02

Meaney, Michael, McGill University, Montreal, Canada reported Buffalo News, 7/19/00

Hopper, Ian. AP News report, Buffalo News, 7/l4/2000

Reinesch, Dr. June, Column *Kinsey Report*, Buffalo News, November 1, l992

Merrill, Mike, Buffalo News, September 13, 1991

Darrach, Forest Jacqueline, co-author Alan Guttmacher, Institute Study of Reproductive Health, reported in Buffalo News, 12/11/92

Lloyd J. Thomas, PHD, Psychologist, Schenectady Daily Gazette, 4/12/02

DeVaus, David, LaTrobe University in Melbourne, Australia, reported by AP in Schenectady Daily Gazette, 10/5/02

American College of Obstetricians Annual Meeting. Reported in the Schenectady Daily Gazette, 5/1/01

Quote from Commencement address by Wm. Raspberry at UNC at Chapel Hill, NC—reported in Schenectady Daily Gazette 6/17/02

Medco Health, AP report, Schenectady Daily Gazette, 9/19/02

Brown, Sarah, Director National Campaign to Prevent Teen Pregnancy, AP News Report, Schenectady Daily Gazette 9/26/02

University of Minnesota, Los Angeles Medical Center, University of California at Davis, Mount Sinai School of Medicine, AP Release Schenectady Daily Gazette, 11/11/02

The Lancet Medical Journal, reported in Schenectady Daily Gazette, 4/27/01

Parker, Kathleen, Columnist, Orlando Sentinel, reported in Niagara Falls Gazette 5/17/99

Audio/Video Works

Peck, Scott, M.D., Tape on Self-love vs. Self-esteem, Simon & Schuster Audioworks, New York, N.Y., 1989

Potter, Dr. Jesse, *The Touch Film*, Sterling Products, 500 N. Dearborn St., Chicago, Ill.

Silverstone, Robert, Dr., and Rhonda Wise, "What Kids Want To Know About", Children's Television Workshop, Lincoln Place, New York, NY—shown Channel 17 (Buffalo, NY) 5/13/92

Interviews/Lectures

Casarjean, Robin, Talk on Forgiveness, given at Hospice Conference, Hilton Hotel, Buffalo, NY, Fall, 1990

Franz, Thomas, M. D., professor of Counseling Psychology at State University of New York at Buffalo, (personal interview) 9/21/92

Reports

American Medical Assn Study, "Wellness Today", Special Supplement to Health and Healing, April 1992.

Committee of the White House, *Conference on Childhood and Youth*, March of 1950

Friends & Lovers in the College Years, formulated by the Committee on the College Student Group for the Advancement of Psychiatry, Published by Mental Health Material Center, New York, NY, 1983

Geist, Valerius, *Children's Initiative, Synopsis of Interim Finding*, Child Abuse Center: report from SCAA, 1 Columbia Place, Albany, NY

Pupura, Dominick, M.D. editor of "Brain Research", professor of Albert Einstein Medical College

Men Have Babies Too: A Guide for Fathers-to-Be, March of Dimes Brochure, Greater New York, 1992

National Council of Juvenile and Family Court Judges, 1989, Report of the California Task Force on Self-esteem, published by the Chamber of Commerce of California, 1990.

978-0-595-39337-4
0-595-39337-3